Tender

Tender

The Imperfect Art of Caring

Penny Wincer

CORONET

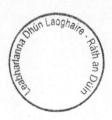

First published in Great Britain in 2020 by Coronet
An imprint of Hodder & Stoughton
An Hachette UK company

2

Copyright © Penny Wincer 2020

A CIP catalogue record for this title is available from the British Library

Hardback ISBN 9781529331219
eBook ISBN 9781529331233

Typeset in Sabon MT by Hewer Text UK Ltd, Edinburgh
Printed and bound in Great Britain by Clays Ltd, Elcograf S.p.A.

Hodder & Stoughton policy is to use papers that are natural, renewable
and recyclable products and made from wood grown in sustainable
forests. The logging and manufacturing processes are expected to
conform to the environmental regulations of the country of origin.

Hodder & Stoughton Ltd
Carmelite House
50 Victoria Embankment
London EC4Y 0DZ

www.hodder.co.uk

For my mother Christine Wincer, who wanted me
to learn from what she had been through.

And for Arthur and Agnes,
who continue to teach me every day.

Contents

Foreword

5th April 2020

As I have been reading through the final proofs of this book, the world has changed. Though we all hope that the extreme situation we find ourselves in is temporary, it is also impossible to ignore. Three weeks ago, in a 24-hour period, like so many carers and disabled people, I lost almost all my support overnight. Support built painstakingly through years of meetings, arguments, form filing and hope crumbled in an instant. Some of the interviewees in these pages have retained some of their paid carers for now, but many have lost most or all support and are now caring for their family members 24 hours a day.

Even more worrying than the extreme demands being put on unpaid carers is the way disabled people are experiencing this crisis. The British Medical Association has warned that if there is a lack of ventilators, a frailty score will be used, which will mean people without any co-existing conditions will be given priority if difficult choices need to be made. The Corona Virus Bill heard in parliament will downgrade the responsibility of Local Authorities from providing social care to whoever is eligible to where it is "reasonably" possible for the next two years. The same goes for fulfilling EHCPs (Education and Healthcare Plans). It is only those with the highest needs who currently receive social care and have EHCPs in place and this bill will allow those needs to be ignored. The leaders of the major disability charities in the UK have said they "fear that the Bill's proposed withdrawal of rights and safeguards for disabled people requiring care and support, will put those in greatest need at greatest risk."[1] Whether or not any of these measures get used, it has been made loud and clear that in a crisis, the rights of disabled people are on unstable ground.

Carers and disabled people are well placed to deal with the emotional effects, many of whom have already spent years coming to terms with isolation and a lack of control. Many are also accustomed to the mental gymnastics required to adjust to yet another difficult situation. As I reread the proofs, I was reminded of the challenges that many carers and disabled people are facing every single day and just how well they handle them. But I also felt it was impossible finish the book without acknowledging the pressure that we are all now under. We can do difficult things, that we know. But we also need the support of the wider community more than ever.

When this crisis is over, let us hope that all those who have never experienced isolation before, those who have never had to rely so heavily on their community before and who will be able to return to their lives with freedom of movement, jobs and access to education, will remember those for whom this has always been difficult. That perhaps society will retain some empathy. That we will remember how we clapped for the NHS when we next go to the polls, that we will remember how it feels to be housebound and reliant on other to bring us necessities, that we will remember how flexible working allowed us to retain jobs in the most challenging of times. Because for many disabled people and carers this is how life has always been. Perhaps we can even hope that this crisis will lead to positive change.

Introduction

Becoming a carer

The realisation that my now 10-year-old son Arthur was struggling emerged over a very long period of time. Small things slowly pieced together that left me feeling uneasy or like a paranoid mother. When he was around 18 months old, I was speaking on the phone to a girlfriend in Australia and she excitedly asked what he was interested in these days. My mind went blank. And then I thought, 'that's not right is it?', that I had no answer to her question. Arthur loves going to the playground, I said after a moment. But in my mind I was thinking, well he used to like the playground. But does he now? My thoughts went to the previous day when he had screamed when I suggested he did anything other than go down the slide again and again. Then there was the time in the Science Museum when we received dirty looks because he only wanted to repeatedly remove the toy boats from the water tanks instead of playing with them in the 'correct' way. At the time I thought the other parents were just being uptight and bossing their children around. If they weren't hovering over their child's every move, I thought, maybe their kids would choose to play differently too. And then there was the time I now look back on as the first obvious full sensory meltdown that had us both sobbing and clambering to find our buggy in an over-crowded, stiflingly hot playgroup.

It was all so slow and creeping that by the time an official diagnosis of autism was given, when Arthur was three, I had already become accustomed to the idea that we were going to have to do everything a bit differently. I hadn't driven in the car with him for a year after his sister Agnes had been born, just after he turned two. He couldn't seem to cope with the combina-tion of being strapped in along with Agnes making any kind of noise, and he would scream and thrash, and she would then cry and on it went in an infinite loop. So no car. I told the nursery where he was starting to do short half days that this was my solution, no car, and they told me I couldn't live life just avoiding things. Even then I thought how ignorant that was. Now our life is full of adjustments and avoidances to support Arthur's needs.

Even though I was more than ready to accept the diagnosis when it came, desperate for any help possible, it still loomed large and overwhelming with an impossible number of question marks attached to it. In some ways Arthur seemed joyful, delighted with the sensory world, and was the sweetest, most affectionate boy I could imagine (yes, autistic people can be very affectionate). But he was also incredibly distressed a lot of the time, easily over-whelmed, barely able to communicate even non-verbally let alone verbally, and impossible to engage in anything other than very high-energy play. At three he loved dancing around the kitchen to opera. We joked that with Arthur it was like living in an opera, all high drama and extreme emotions, nothing temperate or in-between. No calm engagement or quiet play. It was squeals of delight or wails of agony. By the time we had a diagnosis, it had been a year-and-a-half since his sister was born and I had yet to leave them alone in a room together, even for a moment. I couldn't trust him around her. Not until she was old enough to run away if she needed to. I would drag the bouncer into the bathroom so I could watch her while I had a shower, or wait until after they were in bed at night. They had separate rooms and I had elaborate ways in which I could manage bedtimes, which mostly meant Agnes was always the one who had to wait.

We were learning to adapt to our way of family life. I was beginning to piece together the hundreds of strategies we needed to get through an ordinary day. Like any parent with very young children I would be flat out from start to finish, and only when I collapsed in bed at night would the thoughts all finally descend on me. A disabled child. A non-speaking child, so dependent on me. Me, who had no guidance from anyone and had never been a parent before. I was expected to know what to do and how to deal with it. I had absolutely no idea what I was doing.

And yet, I had been here before. I had been a carer before. The feeling of claustrophobia that hit me at night that I so desperately wanted to escape was not just because I had no idea what I was doing as a parent but because I *did* know what it was like to be a carer. I had already done this and I couldn't do it again, I thought to myself. But I am doing it again. This time it was my little boy. Like so many new mothers, the only person who I truly thought could help me in my situation was the one I had already cared for and the one who had died.

My first experience of caring

My mother had her first panic attack when I was 11 years old; I remember it clearly. I grew up in Australia, and that day we were moving to a house on a farm on the outskirts of Melbourne that my parents had built. My mother had worked so hard project-managing the build, but still she was reluctant to move and leave behind our old life. I had taken the day off school to help out. I can still picture her laid across the backseat of our family car, gasping for air. She thought she was having a heart attack. Dad drove the three of us to the hospital. We waited a few hours while they did ECGs and other tests. In the end we were told it was a panic attack. It was the first time I had heard that term and I had no idea then it would come to dominate the next couple of years living in that isolated house on top of a hill.

The move to the farm drew a clear line through my childhood which I can look back on now and see as before Mum was ill, and after. Before had been practically idyllic. She loved being a mother and it showed. My dad travelled for work for months at a time and my mother held everything together at home, and was amazing at it. She was beautiful, warm and kind, had many friends, cooked delicious food, loved spending time in the garden and seemed to thrive on being needed as a mother. At one point my brothers and I were at three different schools, each with completely different Saturday activities, and yet she never seemed harried to me or at all resentful of how time-consuming it all must have been. She was just so good at it all.

Over the couple of years we lived on the farm, my mother became more and more isolated. When my parents decided to separate and we moved with my mum back to town, I thought things would improve for her. At the farm I had been dependent on her, needing her to drive me the few miles to the school bus stop each day. The car seemed to bring on panic attacks and she was terrified of getting in it each day. The house was large and we rattled around in it. She often asked me to come and sleep in her room while Dad was away; she was afraid of being alone. So when we left the farm when I was 13, despite my parents' divorce I thought it was the beginning of things getting better. But things seemed to spiral downwards very quickly. She would stay in bed for days at a time, drinking and locking herself away in the house, rarely seen by anyone.

She would start to cook a meal, then fall asleep before she had finished, so I would rescue it from burning. Other days she wouldn't cook at all. She started giving me money to catch the tram down to the supermarket to do the shopping. I realised the only washing getting done was once a week when the cleaner came, so I started doing more of it in between so I had a clean uniform to wear. I made sure I did my homework, turning up to school and pushing letters and notes to sign in front of her when necessary. My eldest brother Ashley had been at boarding school while were living at the farm and had decided to stay on even though we were back in town. My other brother Pip got himself to school but didn't bother with his homework – since no one was checking – and spent a lot of time with friends. Periodically Mum would become so low that she would go as an inpatient to a private psychiatric clinic; with my dad now living in the US, we would either go and stay with friends, or a babysitter would come and stay with us. When she was at home I would sit by her bed each evening, holding her hand while she cried and told me she wanted to die. Some days she would scream in a drunken rage at me for not being supportive enough. Other times she would beg my forgiveness for not being the mother she had been before. Each day I would catch the train to school and carry on as if our life was just the same as it had always been.

She remained in this cycle of deep depression, drinking, crisis, hospitalisation, improvement and back again for many years. She had good times, too. But somehow they would make the bad times even harder. We would have our loving, warm and gener-ous mother back, showing up. And then she would be gone again. I learned to take care of myself, as did my brothers. And I learned to take care of her. Checking on her each morning before leaving for school and coming home each day, sitting by her bed and listening to her worries. Learning to know when she was not in her right mind and to dismiss the harsh and ugly things she would say to me. Reminding myself that she was ill and not cruel. Softening her difficulties by not asking anything of her and not revealing any of my feelings when it became clear that if she thought I was struggling she only got worse.

As the years went by, I became accustomed to the way our relationship had settled into something else. Mother and daughter who loved each other very much but for whom the balance was always going to be flipped. It would be me checking up on her, making sure she was ok and if there was anything she needed, not the other way around. We had open and very honest conversations when she was capable of them. I learned a lot from her about how I did and did not want to live my life, from her capacity for empathy and non-judgment of all those whom she encountered as a mental health patient. I may not have been able to rely on her but I loved her so much. I thought we would continue forever in this cycle of good times and bad.

Eleven years almost to the day after she had that first panic attack, my mother hanged herself. I was 22. I heard the news late at night in London, where I had moved to only a few weeks before, having just finished university. As I lay in bed awake that night, trying to force myself to sleep before the long flight back to Melbourne, such a strange feeling took over me. It was shock, yes, but it was something else too. I was 14 when my mother had made her first suicide attempt; I had been waiting for this call for years. Waiting for it and dreading it – and now the waiting was over. Amidst the shock and the acute pain I felt at the permanence of it, a part of me deep inside released a breath I'd been holding for years. It was no longer my job to look after her.

Thirteen years later I recognised the panic I felt as it became clear that Arthur was going to be very dependent on me. Again, I was lying in the dark, forcing myself to try to sleep. This time, far from being over, it was just beginning. This time I was no longer the child who needed to care for her mother but a mother who felt practically like a child, so little did I know about how to support my autistic son. There would be no private clinics this time, no one sweeping in to help during a crisis. Thanks to private health insurance my mother had been able to afford a psychiatrist, inpatient stays when she was at her worst, and a paid carer who would come to the house a few times a week to check on her, so that my brothers and I weren't shouldering the responsibility entirely on our own.

This time it was all my responsibility. It was becoming clear to me that my marriage was going to end and I had no mother to call for back up, no extended family who weren't thousands of miles away. As Arthur's father and I settled into a new routine with me as the children's main carer, taking a break every other weekend while he spent time with them, I knew I was going to have to figure a lot of this out on my own. In my area, the NHS offered almost nothing in terms of advice and support for a developmental disability. Arthur was initially given four speech therapy sessions, and the following year another four. I was told there was no funding for occupational therapy for autistic children. I was expected to support him myself until he was school age, despite everything I read saying that early support was vital to an autistic child's development.

I felt I might implode under the pressure. It felt insurmountable. I had done this before and it was so hard. The situation was very different, and yet I felt a similar sense of being out of my depth in holding someone else's wellbeing in my hands. I had and still have so many fears. How would I look after myself, while looking after my son's high needs? What if the pressure became too much?

I had seen what can happen to a person when they struggle with anxiety, depression and addiction. We might be better at talking about mental health than we were 20 years ago, when my mother felt like a pariah, but I had seen the ugly, painful mess up close. My mother had lost everything. And I had lost her bit by bit from that first panic attack to the day she died. Her illness had dominated half of my life with her. At times it had made her completely incapable of being there for us. Looking at my children in those early days after Arthur's diagnosis, I worried about how little support I had. How was I going to cope? What if I ended up like my mother?

What is a carer?

In the UK it is estimated that at any one time there are 8 million people caring for loved ones.[2] According to the Carers Trust, a carer is defined as anyone who cares, unpaid, for a friend or family member, who due to illness, disability, mental health problem or addiction, cannot cope without their support.

We live in a society that doesn't speak much about caring for someone else. If we do speak of it, it's often about caring for elderly family members. Our fear of death and disability rears up and we keep conversations to the relatively safe bounds of inevitable old age. But disability and chronic illness can happen at any time of life and on-going support may be needed for decades. When I started searching out information about being a carer, so much was centred around the assumption that it won't be for very long. But in fact many of us will be supporting some-one else for the rest of our lives. In the UK 8% of children and 19% of working-age adults are disabled,[3] and many of those people require on-going support from a family member. We are living longer than ever before and this means that the likelihood of us requiring care has increased.

Many people don't easily identify as carers. They may be parents or partners, siblings or children, and they may be doing it alongside other commitments such as full-time work, raising other children or going to school. They may be caring from a distance, for short amounts of time, or it might be live-in, 24 hours a day, or anything between the two; the breadth of carer experience is wide and extremely varied. It might be supporting a child born with a life-long disability or genetic condition. It could be supporting someone with a chronic illness such as multiple sclerosis, arthritis or heart disease, with a degenerative condition such as motor neuron disease, a mental health problem like severe depression, or following an accident or serious illness. Caring responsibilities may increase slowly over many years, with adjustments gradually being made as a family member gets older and acquires common chronic illnesses of old age, or it could be very sudden and become intense overnight. Some caring situations are temporary, with a loved one eventually recovering much of their previous independence – or dying. Others are decades long.

The kinds of support carers provide vary so much that it's no wonder many don't identify with the word. Many people associate caring with intensive personal care such as helping someone in and out of bed, bathing them, helping them use the toilet, feeding them and dressing them. While this is true for many, the support an unpaid carer provides can go far beyond that. Here are just a few examples of the kind of support that many of the people I have interviewed for this book are providing: legal advocacy to access an appropriate education; co-ordination of different medical teams and interventions; administering medication and tube feeding throughout the day and night; carrying out physiotherapy, occupational therapy and speech therapy; finding, buying and maintaining appropriate equipment such as mobility aids and specialist beds and hoists; adjusting the house to meet the needs of the person they're supporting; adjusting the rest of the family's activities and needs around that person; advocating for them to gain access to public spaces; providing financial support; being a companion, cook, driver and source of emotional support. It can also be a child keeping a household running while their parent is unable to, or being there to pick up the pieces when an alcoholic falls off the wagon, or attending endless meetings trying to get teachers who should know better to understand the needs of a child with a developmental disability. It can mean becoming more of an expert in a certain condition than most medical practitioners, especially when you are supporting someone who isn't fully able to advocate for themselves.

Access to paid carers, personal assistants and respite brings with it a whole other set of issues. Many people with access to social-care funding struggle to find quality paid carers for the hourly rate that they are allowed to pay. Funds sit languishing in accounts, only to go straight back to the local authority when they go unused. Paid carers may quit if the situation is too challenging for them. Respite centres and overnight care that's on offer locally might be completely inappropriate for the person you're supporting. Handovers between paid staff and unpaid carers can involve paperwork equivalent to that of a medical professional. And that's after all the advocacy it takes to secure any funding. In order to get some social care in place, many find themselves in court proceedings, keeping records that even trained medical staff would find challenging – and all while supporting a family member at the same time.

To be a carer is often to be a medical advocate, therapist, an expert in education law, a finance expert, a nurse, psychologist and, above all else, a care co-ordinator who must be in touch with every medical, social-care and educational institution that your loved one is in need of. Supporting someone else goes far beyond the time you spend in their company, physically and emotionally assisting them.

The price of caring

Caring for someone we love is not unusual. It is the most human thing to do. Yet unpaid care comes at a high price. A survey conducted by Carers UK and the Jo Cox Loneliness Commission in 2018 found that eight out of ten carers feel lonely or socially isolated as a result of their caring role.[4] While carers are supporting and improving the lives of loved ones, holding families together and saving the government billions of pounds by making such a huge contribution, they lose social connections. Half of all carers struggle to get out of the house enough to socialise. A third say they find it very difficult to speak to anyone about their role as a carer, and that has made them feel isolated.

Finances can be very strained by a caring role, with many people having to reduce work hours in order to support a loved one, or give up work altogether; Carer's Allowance is the lowest of all benefits in the UK. People who have been caring for more than 15 years, and those providing more than 35 hours a week of support, are the most likely to experience financial difficulties. There are currently over 1.3 million people in the UK providing more than 50 hours of support a week to a family member.[5] 40% of disabled children are living in poverty,[6] with 1 in 6 disabled children regularly going without food and 1 in 4 going without specialist equipment and adaptations.[7] This may be largely due to the fact that a disabled child may not be able to access typical childcare settings, making it extremely difficult for parents to continue working. Lack of flexible working from employers, combined with the number of medical appointments a child may have to attend, can mean a parent has no choice but to give up work. 84% of mothers of disabled children do not work at all, compared with 39% of mothers of non-disabled children. Because of the gender pay gap, it is more likely to be women who give up paid hours of work for unpaid caring responsibilities. This in turn has a knock-on effect on how well they are able to save for their own retirement.

Although men are increasingly taking on unpaid caring responsibilities, the majority are still carried out by women; worldwide, women are still doing 75% of all unpaid work.[8] Not only are women more likely to die from Alzheimer's disease, they are two-and-a-half times more likely to be providing intense 24-hour care of someone with dementia. Overall, 58% of all carers are women, but that rises to 72% when it comes to those in receipt of Carer's Allowance[9] (which means they care for someone for more than 35 hours a week).

Then there are the health consequences of providing high levels of care to someone else. 61% of carers in the UK say they have suffered physical ill health as a direct result of their caring responsibilities and 72% say their mental health has suffered.[10] Carers are more likely than non-carers to live with chronic illness or disability themselves[11] and anxiety levels in carers is twice as high as the general population.[12] Perhaps, given all this, it is unsurprising that carers report much lower levels of happiness then the general population – 4.5 out of 10 compared with an average of 7.5.[13]

Carers are facing insurmountable pressures. In the UK these pressures have only increased in the past 10 years, as austerity measures have slashed NHS and social-care budgets, making it ever harder for disabled people to access support, and putting more responsibility onto the shoulders of family and friends. There is a very high price to pay for austerity. It goes far beyond the day-to-day difficulties of supporting a loved one, stretching into the future with poverty and poorer mental and physical health. This has been accompanied by the demonisation of disabled people in mainstream media, with stories of benefit fraud and a use of language that implies the cost of disabled people comes to the detriment of everyone else. In fact, disability-related benefits have the lowest rates of any benefit fraud in the UK.[13]

It is impossible to look at these figures and not wonder why the realities of caring isn't a topic talked about more openly and widely. It is likely to be something most of us will do in our lifetime, and the number of carers is increasing year on year. With living longer than ever comes an increase in how long we may spend living with a disability or chronic condition. Yet so many of us find it difficult to discuss the support we provide a loved one, even with close family and friends. Politicians make speeches on social care that centre entirely on the elderly, as if great swathes of working-age disabled people and disabled children do not exist. As if providing care is something we only need to do for people at the very end of their lives.

It can take years for someone who provides support for another to even identity as a carer. This means that by the time they reach out for help, they are often already isolated and in dire need of support. Though much more is needed from government institutions in terms of financial and physical help, there is a wider issue here that encompasses all of society. How do we create an environment where carers aren't afraid to speak about what is happening? How do we normalise the role of carers in mainstream culture, so that our stories are shared and heard?

How do we discuss disability and chronic illness in a way that acknowledges how normal and prevalent these experiences are?

Coming to terms with a diagnosis

As I came to terms with my son's diagnosis, and the early panic of finding ways to support his needs began to subside, I was left with many more questions. I knew that I must find a way to live as full a life as possible, that I *would* find a way. If my experiences with my mother had taught me anything, it was that I was capable of much more than I could imagine. But how do we live our lives as carers when we have so many financial, physical and emotional constraints on us? As I searched and read and explored ideas, I noticed that things were changing for me. Though my life on the surface looked pretty challenging – as a single parent running a business, supporting my son's high needs with never quite enough sleep – I realised that, actually, I was pretty happy most of the time. Yet nothing significant had changed.

When my son was small I could only picture a happy future in which he was talking, had friends and didn't struggle to do the most basic things. And here I was, in a reality that I assumed would make me utterly miserable, actually pretty damn happy. Currently at 10 years old, Arthur only uses a small amount of verbal language, he doesn't have friends his own age in the traditional sense, he can't play any games that involve rules, or waiting or turn taking, unless heavily supported by an adult. He goes to a specialist school and requires one-to-one support to keep him safe, and though we experience some fairly extreme challenges some days, I honestly think I am a happy person. I would have struggled to believe this was possible in the months after diagnosis, when imagining a future with a child as disabled as my son seemed the bleakest prospect in the world. Part of that is naturally adjusting to the challenges. But it goes beyond simply getting used to them.

When I looked at my son and decided that I was determined we would have a wonderful life, no matter whether he spoke a word or could be independent, something changed. It hasn't been an easy shift. At times I feel I am fighting against a tidal wave of cultural pressure to be miserable with the circumstances in which I have found myself.

And yet I am in an incredibly privileged position as a carer. I am a white, middle-class, non-disabled woman with a university education and a flexible career. If I find it difficult supporting a disabled child, you can bet that poverty, poor access to education, institutional racism, insecure housing, childhood trauma, learning difficulties, disability and chronic illness, gender violence, and language and cultural barriers all make accessing support *far* more difficult. When I was supporting my mother as a teenager, she could afford a paid carer for a few hours a few times a week, had insurance that covered hospitalisation, owned her own home and was not in danger of being evicted. All of these things made my life much easier as a young carer, and they are things many people do not have access to.

In order for the lives of disabled people and those who support them to be the best they can be, to have access to the things in life that we all deserve to have access to, our stories cannot remain in the shadows. Right now, caring and disability are represented in mainstream culture as either pitiable and miserable, or as stories to inspire others. But the truth is that we are just ordinary people, doing our very best to support someone we love. If we can open a door to that world for others to see, perhaps that conversation with our friends will become a little easier. Our loved ones, doctors and teachers will understand our fears a little better. Other family members will see the pressures we are under. As a society we all need to get better at reaching out to those who need more support. No more so than those who are too busy, too unable to recognise how they have been ignoring their own needs, who will likely burn to the ground looking after someone else before they ask for help.

In my experiences supporting my mother and now my son, I have had my eyes opened to the most beautiful and the ugliest of human emotions. I have been racked with fear and guilt, resentful of what has been asked of me, seen the most incredible joy, loved harder than I could have imagined and picked myself up sobbing from the floor more times than I can count.

Feeling less alone

It is not the point of this book to minimise the acute difficulties that so many of us face as carers. This book will not solve problems around getting accessible housing or finding appropriate paid support so you can return to work. It will not help your disabled child sleep (sorry) or reduce the mountains of paperwork that are piling up around you. But I do hope that, like me, you find the stories of other carers make you feel less alone. Less like the only one awake at 2am. Less afraid of speaking up about what is happening behind closed doors. More able to see how well you're handling a very difficult situation, and more able to see the joy in a life that you didn't imagine you would have.

This is the book I needed someone to press into my hands as a teenager who didn't know the word 'carer' applied to me. It is the book I desperately searched for as a parent to a newly diagnosed child. It contains only a fraction of some of the hidden stories of people walking down similar paths, many of whom are thriving. I have been driven by a deep curiosity to understand all that has happened to me as a carer.

I wanted to know why it was so difficult for many of us to speak openly about our experiences. What was behind the intense perfectionism that I saw rising up in me as I started my journey as the parent to a disabled child. How our experiences as carers are shaped by a culture around us that persists in speaking of disability or illness as the biggest tragedy that can befall a person. How can we adjust our expectations when our life goes in a direction far beyond our control? How can we demand and get the rest we need? What can we do with the intense and difficult feelings that come up? What does it mean to grieve for a person before they have died? How do we keep putting one foot in front of the other when we are on our knees, shattering into a thousand pieces, certain that we won't be able to keep going for another day, let alone years?

It is not possible to capture in one book the full breadth of experiences that carers face. Not every scenario, condition or relationship is covered. But in the conversations that drew me to write about other carers, I found that although we each may face some very different challenges, there is much that we have in common. Just as my experience supporting my mother has shaped the carer I am to my son, the act of caring goes beyond the strict confines of particular relationships – and there is much we can gain from each other's experiences.

You won't find here information or instructions on the more practical aspects of supporting an ill or disabled loved one, such as applying for Carer's Allowance, the best home adaptations for someone with limited mobility or advice on how to advocate for your child in an educational tribunal, for instance. I'll leave that to the experts in each field and you'll find a list of resources at the end of the book that may be helpful.

You'll also see that in many cases I do not list or sometimes even mention the specific kinds of support that some carers are providing their loved one, outside of explaining the disability or impairments that person has. This is to protect the privacy of the people involved. I think you'll also find that it is unnecessary for us to know the details – such as if a person requires assistance bathing or not – to understand and grasp the essence of the support someone is providing, and the way that has impacted on their life.

Where it's relevant and I have permission, it's included. Where it's either irrelevant, or the person involved has decided it's too private, it isn't included.

Each of the carers I have interviewed have the permission of the person whom they support to share their story and, in many cases where it was possible and appropriate, I also spoke to the person receiving support. Where the person being cared for is a child, I have allowed parents to make the decision as to what details are mentioned, although I have excluded any details in direct relation to personal care such as toileting, whether it came up or not. In some cases names have been changed for privacy.

Although being a carer can mean many different things, including supporting someone from a distance, for just a few hours a week, or for a short intense period at the end of life, I have chosen to focus on the stories and experiences of those who are in it – for the most part – for the long haul; those who have been a carer for many years or who have many years still ahead of them. Some are supporting a loved one through an inevitable and slow decline which will end in death. Some are supporting a loved one who will hopefully have a long life ahead of them, but who will not manage without their support. Each scenario has its own complications, fears and worries. Each relationship between supporter and supported is unique in both its challenges and its love.

The night after I gave birth to Arthur, I stood holding him in my arms in the stiflingly hot hospital ward, showing him London stretched before me. Big Ben and the Houses of Parliament, river boats going by all lit up with Christmas parties, people hurrying across Westminster Bridge in a light snow. He had been early and was tiny, but just big enough that he didn't require special care. I looked down at his little face, thinking of that moment at his birth when the midwives realised he wasn't breathing. He was whipped away to the resuscitation table across the room, and after only a short time began to cry. Loving a baby this much was a big risk when there were no guarantees in life. I had a sudden and overwhelming feeling of not wanting to know what the future held. For now he was safe and well in my arms and nothing else mattered, I thought to myself. I'm glad I didn't know that night what we were in for, he and I. I don't think I would have believed I could handle it. But every day I wake up and cuddle Arthur and help him through his day, and I am handling it, just like the millions of other carers doing the same. And it is worth it to be part of this world that I would have never known. It is worth it for his love.

CHAPTER I

Why is it So Hard to Talk About Caring?

'I absolutely failed at being the perfect caregiver for Rayya when she was sick and dying . . . I decided it was my job to take care of her, and I intended to do it with excellence, honour, patience, skill, spirituality, grace and unconditional love. Well friends: I failed at it. Again and again, I failed. I was overcome by exhaustion, by my own grief, by anger at her for being an uncooperative and ungrateful patient, by resentment of anyone who disagreed with me about her care, by anger at God for letting her die. I fell apart. I fell short.'

Elizabeth Gilbert, author

My mother and I were in her car together, side by side. It hadn't been long since I'd finished school, and with my brand-new driver's licence I had taken on most of the driving. She was in a bad mood; I felt a fight coming on. That familiar prickle was in the air as her words became curter, snappier and more defensive. I don't remember what we had initially been talking about, perhaps it was my impending year abroad. But out of nowhere, as so many of these arguments seemed to begin, she told me that her old friend, whom we'd had lunch with the previous day, had been on the phone to her that morning complaining about me. She told me this friend had thought I had treated her (my mum) terribly, that I was short with her, impatient and rude. My mum practically spat the words at me. 'See!' she said to me, feeling somewhat vindicated that she wasn't the only one who thought I was rude and impatient with her.

I was shocked. I had known this friend of my mother's all my life. My cheeks burned with shame as I let Mum continue her rant. We were just about to pull up in front of our house when I finally put some words together. 'And where has she been, Mum?' I asked. 'Where has she been the last five years?' I turned off the engine and said I needed to go to the shops quickly to get something and that I would be right back. After my mother got out of the car and went inside, I drove down our quiet suburban street and found a spot to pull in. There I sobbed into the steering wheel for 20 minutes.

My mum's friend was right. I had been rude and impatient with her that day at lunch. Over the previous seven years, since I was around eleven years old, I had often been taking care of myself while my mother was in and out of hospital. I had sat by her bedside listening to repeated stories way beyond my years, watched her stay in bed for weeks at a time, tried not to appear too upset when she forgot to turn up for events at school she promised to be at. When I was older, I bought alcohol and cigarettes for her to stop her getting in the car drunk. I lied to her about everything always being fine, knowing that I would only deepen her depression if she thought I wasn't coping. It had all led to me being a bit impatient and rude some days. I would snap and fight back, even if it was clear she was drunk and couldn't control her actions. I would get defensive when she was having good days, wary of allowing her to mother me, knowing it would disappear as soon as she went downhill again. I hated that it made me like that, and the shame of having it pointed out by someone else burned through me.

Whenever my mother went through a crisis during those years, she would go into a private clinic for a two-week stay. I was often told by her psychiatrist not to visit for the first three or four days until the initial crisis (a euphemism for suicide watch) was over, then I would visit every couple of days for the rest of her stay. They were hard visits. At first I would listen to her apologise over and over for letting me down, while I in turn reassured her that she hadn't. Then, as the days ticked by and her mood improved, inevitably when I turned up to see her she would be surrounded by other inpatients, attracted to her warmth and empathetic attitude. Young girls with eating disorders whom she mothered in the absence of their own parents, men and women with a variety of mental illnesses who were drawn to her open and accepting nature. She cared for them, listened to them and validated them in a way she seemed incapable of doing for me. As her daughter, my emotions became too much of a burden for her in her fragile state. But strangers' emotions seemed to be fine. I found myself angry and resentful of the other inpatients for the way they could unburden themselves to my mother. I had learned the hard way that this was something I could no longer do.

I knew it wasn't her fault. I knew she was ill. But I was angry with her anyway. I felt motherless. And then I would feel terrible for thinking about myself when my mum was so ill. How can you be angry at someone who can't control what's happening to them? My feelings of resentment towards her illness spilled over into feeling resentful towards her. I was so ashamed of those feelings that I never spoke about them to anyone. I learned to protect my mother – and others – from how I felt, in order to be strong for her.

To put what is happening to us as carers into words can feel like a betrayal. The illness or impairment isn't happening to us but to someone we love. Where is the space for our own feelings amongst this? I am not alone in having had moments of berating myself for feeling resentful, angry or frustrated. It is the person we are supporting who is working hard to live with physical pain, mental illness or impaired cognition, not us . . . It can feel safer to stay silent about our own inner turmoil. And yet, as carers, while not experiencing the illness or disability, our whole lives may also have been drastically up-ended. We may be facing levels of stress and demands on us that we have never experienced before.

My mother was a brilliant and adored woman who had put us first all our lives. She had spent huge chunks of time solo parenting while my father travelled for work, then full time after their divorce. She made the kind of home that was always welcoming and open to all our friends. She was beautiful, sociable and kind. She was the first to volunteer for anything and had endless supplies of empathy. All of the things that made up my mother now sat incongruously alongside addiction, forgetfulness, stints in private psychiatric hospitals and weeks of being unable to get out of bed. How could I share any of what was happening without people blaming her? Or worse, thinking she was a terrible mother. I wanted to protect her. I didn't want people's opinion to be changed by what she was going through. She was still my mother.

This is true for carers in many situations. Your wife is no less your wife just because you are now having to cut up her food, manage her medication and speak on her behalf at doctors' appointments when she struggles to do so. The same wife who perhaps ran a household, made all the family decisions and raised multiple children. Speaking about the changes that occur in intimate and long-standing relationships can be hard. A betrayal, even. And yet when we fail to say anything, our needs can be lost in amongst their more acute needs. Many carers are flailing and falling to their knees before they realise they can't stay silent any longer.

Whether because of shame surrounding our conflicted feelings or out of protection for those we are caring for, using our voices as carers is a difficult thing to navigate. Carers make up a vulnerable group, but not as vulnerable as those we care for. How can there be room for our own thoughts, feelings and needs when the needs of our loved ones are more extreme? When others depend on us, not only to thrive but often to survive, it can feel right at the time to stay silent. But the costs are high.

There are so many feelings that surface during the act of caring for another person, particularly when the situation spans long periods. Ugly feelings that are hard to acknowledge. Jealousy towards others whose relationship with their parent or partner has remained unchanged by caring. Or jealousy of the freedom that those who are not carers have in choosing what to do with their time, and in living where they wish, or who are unrestricted in the jobs they can take on. Anger at the level of demands that are on you and the lack of support you receive. Guilt every time you leave your loved one in the hands of a paid carer so you can take a break, even when you know you desperately need it. Sadness about the life path you have had to let go of, the opportunities you now must say no to. And although these may be rational feelings, common feelings of those thrown into a caring situation, that you feel these things at all can create intense shame. And yet these feelings arise in the midst of the loving act of caring. It can be hard to admit to ourselves that these feelings exist, let alone to others. Close friends and family may be quite unaware of the physical and emotional toll that our duty as carers is taking on us.

Carers are seven times more likely than the general population to report feeling lonely; they are also twice as anxious.[15] Carers who reported feeling lonely were twice as likely to have worsened mental and physical health than carers who did not feel lonely. In the USA, 40% to 70% of carers have clinically significant symptoms of depression and around half of those meet the criteria for major depression.[16] Apart from being able to take regular breaks from caring, the next most important thing that carers report needing, to help combat loneliness, is more understanding from society. We will never have more understanding if we remain silent and hidden from the world.

Not identifying with the word 'carer'

Sarah Roberts' son Oscar was diagnosed with Down's syndrome shortly after his birth seven years ago. When we met, she described the vivid image that came into her mind as the doctor told her the news. It was of a sad old woman and a middle-aged son, dressed badly in childlike clothing with a dodgy haircut. They're holding hands and shuffling around a shopping centre. The pain that gripped her in that moment was the fear of becoming that woman. She doesn't know where the image came from, but it was what immediately came to her mind when she heard the words 'Down's syndrome' and 'life-long disability'. It's an image that she feels is so far from the life she now leads that it has spurred her on to share her life on social media. She hopes that for someone else out there who receives a surprise diagnosis, it will be the image of her son and the full lives they lead as a family – the challenges and the joys included – that they will associate with the disability.

Not identifying with the word 'carer' is something that comes up a lot in the conversations I have with others raising disabled children or living with disabled partners or parents. Some have told me outright they don't like the word and its connotations. A 'carer' is a sad figure to many – someone leading an isolated life in service to another, someone with no economic power, taking on gruelling physical work to care for a person utterly dependent on them. With disability and caring so often hidden away, I wasn't particularly surprised to hear so many people say they didn't identify with the word. Caring is something other people do. Many people told me they were simply being a parent, a wife, a husband or a son, just with some extra responsibilities thrown in. I would have said the same back when I was 14. I didn't know that as a teenager with a mother who sometimes didn't leave her bedroom for weeks on end, that in taking on her responsibilities, as well as making sure she was safe, eating and alive, I was not just being a daughter, I was being a young carer.

When I spoke to Sally Derby, she said using the word carer to talk about her husband is challenging. Sally has multiple sclerosis and a visual impairment, and was a secondary school teacher for many years until she felt she couldn't manage it any longer. She said that the word carer often gave people the image of someone cleaning up bodily fluids and that it can also diminish other parts of your relationship in other people's eyes – the carer part being what people remember. But that's not how their relationship feels at all, she says. They are first and foremost husband and wife. But he also provides care.

In the UK, approximately one in eight us at any one time is providing support for someone chronically ill or disabled.[17] Over a lifetime, almost all of us will be a carer at some point. Carers are next to you in the queue at the coffee shop, playing with their kids in the park and in your meetings at work. But to admit to being a carer brings with it many fears for some. Fear of being pitied. Fear of not getting the job if you mention it in an interview. Fear of becoming more isolated than you already are. Fear of losing other parts of your identity, swallowed up by the enormity of the role as well as the low status that it holds in our society. And, above all else, using the word carer will mean admitting openly that someone you love cannot manage without your support. It means facing up to their illness or disability and possibly their death. And that can be a difficult process for many, no matter the relationship they have with the person they support.

Although the gender divide between carers is gradually shrinking, caring is still very much seen to be something that women do. And like many things that are culturally feminine, caring is massively undervalued in our society, whether it's looking after children or supporting disabled or elderly relatives. Paid carers are among the lowest-paid workers in the UK, usually only receiving minimum wage for what can be physically and emotionally demanding work. Unpaid caring is often viewed in the same light: low-status work done predominantly by women. In the UK it is estimated that the value provided by unpaid carers is around £132 billion. In the USA it is around $470 billion, more than the total spend on paid home care and Medicaid in a year.[18] This figure nearly matches the sales of the world's largest company, Walmart. In the words of Helena Herklots, former Chief Executive of Carers UK, even a small reduction in the number of those able to do unpaid care would be catastrophic to the economy.[19] Despite its lack of status, unpaid caring is absolutely vital.

Yet for carers like Alice Bennett, whose daughter has hydrocephalus and is a wheelchair user, she feels the care she provides is undervalued. People in her life comment on the fact she 'doesn't have to work', when she provides around-the-clock care to her daughter. Alice has found that she is ashamed to admit to people she receives a Carer's Allowance, which is a measly £66 a week. Raya is six years old and needs support with every single aspect of her personal care, and will do for the rest of her life. Her variety of medical needs means she has countless appointments to attend and has had multiple emergency brain surgeries. When Raya finally received a full-time place at a specialist school, Alice felt a huge pressure to get into work. As a single parent with no relatives nearby, she provides all of the support for her daughter outside of school hours, as well as raising another non-disabled daughter. Despite this, Alice enrolled in college and took on a job as a teaching assistant, largely because of the pressure she felt from others to stop living on benefits. But with frequent appointments and hospital admissions, being a working parent of a disabled child can be extremely difficult. Alice discovered quickly that a teaching assistant role was going to leave her burned out and unable to care well enough for her daughters or herself. After our conversation I was left wondering whether anyone critical of her receiving benefits might like to spend a week in her shoes. Or in the shoes of anyone caring for someone else for more than 35 hours a week.

Pity is a topic that comes up again and again in these conversations. Fear of the cocked head, watery eyes and the 'Ahhhh, that must be so hard' comments that often stop us in our tracks before any mention of our role as carers comes up. Our lives may have their challenges, sometimes extremely tough ones, and yet it is pity from others that most carers talk of with horror and sadness. Not only might we be dealing with sleepless nights, endless meetings with doctors and teachers and tending to personal care needs, we must also deal with pity from others about what they imagine our lives must be like. If our roles as carers aren't physically isolating us enough, then it will be the emotional isolation we feel that may tip us over the edge. Pity or sympathy become another reminder that we are alone with our experience. And so it is with self-protection in mind that we may keep the details of our lives to ourselves, until we are in the safe presence of others who share our experiences.

There are some predominant narratives around being a carer that are pervasive, despite being untrue for most. Carers must be either angels, people with capacities and abilities that ordinary humans don't possess, or pitiable, living half-lives dominated by drudgery. Attitudes towards disabled and chronically ill people are still so appalling that to be a carer must either require you to be superhuman or miserable. Online, many disabled people receive abuse, such as being told their mother should have aborted them. Couples where one person is visibly disabled are often told that their relationship is 'unnatural'. Shops, restaurants and public transport, despite there being laws in place, still fail to be wheelchair accessible or provide suitable toilets, meaning disabled people often feel unwelcome in these spaces. Blind people, particularly women, complain of being manhandled in public and then verbally abused when they ask strangers to please not touch them. These daily occurrences not only negatively affect the lives of disabled people but also, to a lesser extent, the people who support them. These common and still frequently socially acceptable attitudes mean it's often easier to keep our mouths shut to those outside our innermost circle.

Cultural depictions of carers often feed into the idea of the angelic, self-sacrificing superhero, which does nothing to help with the guilt that, as real-life caregivers, we often feel we fall short. Particularly prevalent is the heroic carer mother who breezes through her role with only a tiny (and attractive) tear for their child, never for themselves. Think Julia Roberts' depiction of Auggie's mum in the 2018 film *Wonder*. Having cheerfully dedicated her life with no complaints to her son with his severe facial differences and subsequent multiple surgeries, her apparent only bad quality was not paying enough attention to her eldest and non-disabled child. So while she is allowed to be a not-entirely-perfect human being, she is a near-perfect caregiver.

The reality is that for most, caring is exactly like the rest of life. Sometimes wonderful, sometimes terrible and often very ordinary. The cultural conversation often refuses to acknowledge this, instead putting us into camps of either people who are inspiring with life-affirming goodness, or people to be sorry for or to help because of assumed intense suffering. But this creates a massive disservice to the millions of ordinary people in caring roles, and to the people they care for. While it isn't easy being a carer and sometimes it entails extreme difficulties, feeling pitied by others, or being put on a pedestal, just makes the role harder than it needs to be.

In Laura Dorwart's article for *Catapult* magazine, she describes why we so often think carefully before we talk about our caring roles: people's ignorant assumptions.[20] Dorwart's husband Dr Jason Dorwart is a theatre professor and a quadriplegic. She describes the exhausting and awkward reactions she receives, which leave her feeling like she has done her partner a disservice by mentioning it. She finds herself having to reassure the listener that it's no big deal and watch as their eyes 'glaze over with pity' at what they assume – and often voice – must be an awful life. Her husband is now part of what she describes as a collection of stills of disabled people in their mind reduced to that single description of 'quadriplegic' with no individual personality or traits. And as his wife, it's assumed her role as carer is unidirectional. Yet Laura admits to being of very little assistance to her husband at all in comparison to the support he provides her. Caring goes both ways, but in a world conditioned to pity and fear disability, it is unimaginable to many that a relationship between someone in a wheelchair and someone who is not could possibly be balanced and reciprocal.

While some may think it's natural to feel pity for someone in my shoes, the weight of that pity can be extremely heavy. Here is yet another burden carers must carry around with them, and god knows they have enough on their shoulders already. After my mother's suicide when I was 22 years old, I actively avoided mentioning the cause of her death, or the illness that had dominated the last 11 years of her life. I was not ashamed of her. I wasn't avoiding it because it was too painful. I was avoiding it to protect her memory against a world fixed on the narrative that a mother who loved her children would never kill herself. My mother had loved us. And she had fought to live for us for 11 years. Her death from a mental illness did not alter how I knew she felt about my brothers and me. I thought that by not talking about it, by not mentioning the years I spent as one of her carers, I could protect her from a judgmental world. I was also saving myself from uncomfortable, pity-filled conversations in which I always ended up comforting the other person. My mother died too young. I was often sad about that. But her life wasn't a waste and her suicide wasn't selfish. It was a tiring conversation to have. It was easier not to speak about it.

These days I'm often working with new clients, and as such the conversations over the lunch table naturally turn to life outside work, family and friends. On any given day I might see the conversation leading to a point at which I would need to mention my son's disability. Some days I just don't have the energy to explain our situation and so subtly steer the subject away. Other days I'm happy to chat about our family situation and its differences; it depends very much on my mood. But at the heart of it is a desire for others to see us as leading whole, fulfilling lives. No one wants to be the family people compare themselves to in a way that says: 'Thank god that's not my life.' So if I do start the conversation, I feel I need to do my best for my son's sake, for my sake and even for the sake of all those families raising neurodivergent children, to give a full picture that's inclusive of the joy and normality that make up the majority of our home life.

When, as Laura Dorwart talks about, people automatically reach for the phrase 'I'm so sorry', we find ourselves needing to prove the value of our lives and the lives of our disabled family members. Sarah Roberts felt so strongly about the pity levelled at her after her son's Down's syndrome diagnosis that she named her blog 'Don't Be Sorry'. 'I'm so sorry' were the first words out of the mouth of the paediatrician who explained that they suspected her son had Down's syndrome, in the hours after his birth. That single phrase sums up much of the problem that disabled people and those caring for them face. Pity, distancing, assumed misery. We spend our time reassuring others that everything is fine, often to such an extent that we can't be open about the times when it is hard and complicated and we may need more support. Our default modes can be set to positive at all times, which is unrealistic for any human. In our need for our lives to be palatable to others in a world where we are pitied and our disabled family members are othered, it's easy to either stay quiet or try to be relentlessly cheerful.

As I write this, we are speeding towards the summer holidays. A tricky time for any working family but most especially for those of us who have children who require structure and routine to keep overwhelm and intense anxiety at bay. As the school year comes to a close and the messy unstructured nature of the seven weeks looms ever closer, my fear and panic start to increase. While my daughter enjoys and needs the rest from the school year, time for play and the kind of boredom that only a long summer can provide, my son will start to flail and panic. I plan as much as I can. But every year the feelings creep up on me.

What kind of mother dreads the summer holidays so much? Does it make me a failure to be afraid of all that open-ended time with my son? How can I possibly provide anything close to what his school can, in terms of predictability and routine, while also meeting my daughter's needs, cooking meals, tidying up and keeping my business running? I chat to other parents about their plans and hear of books they'll be taking on holidays with them, of day trips planned and excursions across the country for impromptu weekends with friends. I sense the excitement many of them feel at the loosening of routines and ditching of the school run. I feel so guilty for not feeling the same. I desperately want to feel that way. But summertime stretches out in front of us like a vast desert to get lost in, and it can feel terrifying.

Other carers have similarly conflicting feelings – the desperate need for breaks followed by the guilt of having to use paid strangers who can't know our loved one's needs as well as we do. The guilt at *having* to get away from someone we love, knowing that they can't get a break from their illness or disability themselves. Some, as the end of life draws nearer, feel both a desperate sense of grief and loss, all the while knowing a part of them will be relieved when it's over.

I hold these two truths in my hands at once. I love being a mother to my son and I can't be his carer all the time without support and breaks. It feels hard and wrong that these two things are true but they are. I want to be a mother who has endless capacity, just as those caring for a parent they love might want to be a dutiful and caring son or daughter, repayment for all those years of care they received as a child. The partners who vowed to love 'in sickness and in health', who desperately want to fulfil that promise.

I want a few sleepless nights not to affect me. I want to always remain calm during a stormy and sudden meltdown. I want to have energy for finding my son activities as he moves listlessly about the house. I wish I didn't beat myself up when he rejects my efforts at play and would rather be on the iPad. I wish I were never fazed by the constant mess created by his sensory-seeking behaviour. Those moments when I'm making pancakes and I turn my back for a second, only to see the flour all over the kitchen. The food that gets thrown for the joy of seeing pink spattered yoghurt along the ceiling, or the patterns chocolate crumbs make when sprinkled over the kitchen chairs. I wish I didn't need breaks from the planning, the anxiety prevention, the hyper-vigilance to keep him physically safe. The times he bolts unexpectedly in the street and I have to make a run and grab before he's hit by a speeding car. Or the careful organising of my week so that I can avoid taking him on an errand that might cause him stress. The military-like planning that even a visit to a friend's house or birthday party involves, assessing all the ways in which he might hurt himself or someone else. Those moments when I make a mistake, misjudge what he can manage and it's my daughter who gets caught up in the meltdown that results.

I'm not always the caregiver I wish I could be. But when I voice these feelings, I'm terrified that people will take that as a reflection of my son, that they will think, 'Ahh, see, having a disabled child is a sad and depressing thing.' I want to scream and rail against this idea because it is not compatible with that other truth that being a mother to Arthur has also been one of the greatest joys of my life. I want people to see both of these things. Our life isn't black and white, good or bad. It is a myriad of all the emotions that humans experience. But I'm not sure that people see that.

'Are you coping?'

When speaking to professionals and service providers, the honest truth about some aspects of care giving can be difficult to say out loud. Away from our loved ones, in the privacy of empty beige clinical rooms, it's difficult to articulate the harder aspects of care in order to receive support. We have to peel away those protective layers and get down to the raw details of what is required of us. Even while facing the reality of being denied support unless we are honest about the difficulties, it can feel shameful to verbally acknowledge them. The armour necessary to move about in the public realm somehow must be shed when faced with an unknown doctor, social worker or local authority employee acting as gatekeeper to much-needed support. To admit to another that you need help raising your own child, or supporting your spouse, can bring with it a deep shame that is hard to describe, something that is explored in more depth in the following chapter.

'Are you coping?' they might say, after I have just described a meltdown that almost ended in me crashing the car when a shoe was thrown at me from the back seat. I don't know how to answer that question. Does the fact we didn't get in an accident that day count as coping? What about when I angrily pulled over and shouted at him? Does that mean I'm not coping? Or because we both calmed down and had a cuddle afterwards, does that mean I am actually coping? I don't know what answer they expect me to be able to give. More help is unlikely to follow either way, whether I admit I'm terrified of falling apart or not. So is it worth being truly honest and vulnerable?

I watch them take notes and I wonder if I have said too much. Or not enough. Do they understand how wonderful he is? Or will they remember him as the kid who almost caused a car accident by throwing a shoe at his mother's head? But if they don't hear the story about the shoe they may not understand why I need some respite hours on the weekends, so that I don't have to take him on errands in the car – something that is too stressful for him. Round and round these thoughts go as I decide what information to reveal and discuss with people I barely know, who will present evidence to other people who will never meet us, to decide whether our situation is worthy of additional support.

When others don't want to hear what's really happening

I have learned over time that not everyone will view our situation as I do. At a meeting at Arthur's first school before he started, I excitedly revealed that he had just called me Mama for the first time, only to see their strained smiles as I realised they thought he was more advanced than that. Friends I haven't seen in a long time ask how he's doing and I say 'great!' 'So he's catching up?' they say with a huge smile and I watch their faces drop as I explain that no, he's not 'catching up', but he can now follow my finger when I point to something. It can be painful and tiring to have to explain to people that something they take for granted is a big deal for us. That the seemingly simple act of pointing can be a skill that some people will struggle with for a lifetime. Our milestones look different. When others don't understand and can't share in the joys of milestones like this, it can be easier just not to share them at all. So we save those conversations for when we are with fellow carers whose faces will instinctively reflect back our joy.

Carers supporting a loved one who is declining may not want to dwell on those losses with others. To have to watch faces drop as they bring news of the latest struggles can add to the burden. Culturally we have become accustomed over the past half century or so to illnesses being cured and diseases eradicated. But medicine can still only slow down the progression of many fatal conditions. Many people don't want to be confronted with the reminder that despite everything humans have achieved, there are times when nothing can stop the inevitable march towards death.

When I spoke to Tatty Bowman about life with her 15-year-old son George, who has a dual diagnosis of Down's syndrome and autism, she was quick to point out what she finds hard to discuss with friends who are not in her situation. Over the last couple of years, George, who is non-speaking, has become quite aggressive towards her for the first time. Tatty suspects it's a mixture of teenage hormones and frustration at needing his mother to tend to so much of his personal care. She confesses that though these incidents are interspersed with lots of love, she is finding it tough that he struggles to be near her and be cared for by her. Looking after all of someone's personal care needs takes energy, love and tenderness, and it's something Tatty is happy to do. She doesn't expect gratitude from him and she knows he can't control his behaviour, so she doesn't blame him. But she is finding it very hard. Two days before this conversation, my son had hit me hard in the face during a meltdown, and while Tatty and I chatted, my fingers went to the still sore spot on the bridge of my nose. It's the kind of conversation that flows easily between two carers who know neither will judge the person for what they have done. But it is a whole different thing to allow someone from outside our world in on the realities of challenging behaviour, where black eyes and pinched skin are an unfortunate but not entirely unusual occurrence.

'Challenging behaviour' is a term that's used by many professionals to describe when a person is unable to remain in control of themselves when they are emotionally disregulated and unable to communicate their needs in other ways. It's not only people with learning difficulties who may experience it, but also people with neurological conditions like dementia, or brain injuries from strokes. For some it can mean hitting, kicking, spitting, scratching and throwing things, for others it is turned inwards and becomes self-harm. For those looking after someone who experiences challenging behaviour, talking about it is extremely difficult.

After the incident that almost broke my nose, I sat on our kitchen floor and cried. Through watery eyes, I tried to reassure Arthur, who had now calmed down, that I was going to be fine, I just needed a minute. But I didn't feel fine. It wasn't just the pain. It was shame. Shame at not being able to help him calm down before he hurt me. Shame at being the kind of mother people either pity or judge. Shame that my efforts at helping him communicate aren't enough. Shame that each professional I tell about that incident will give me a list of things I could be doing better to prevent such a thing happening. Shame at failing to be a good mother.

It's someone else's story too

Historically, disabled people have been actively denied a voice along with many basic human rights, such as the right to education, to reproduce and even the right to live. As a mother I am all too aware of the fact my son has no voice of his own right now, and may or may not ever be able to share his own experiences with the world. So to speak about caring for him is a tricky road to navigate and there will be many who will say I shouldn't speak about it at all. He is both a minor and someone with a learning disability and cannot give me his consent. As his mother I have to think carefully what I share of our life with the outside world (and believe me, much of our life isn't shared). But in a world of social media and blog posts, it isn't surprising that many disabled activists are against non-disabled parents and carers sharing the ins and outs of their child's meltdowns, toileting habits and challenging behaviour. Parental oversharing has the potential to do damage to the millions of disabled people worldwide, who may be having opinions shaped about the quality of their lives thanks to a viral video where a mother cries about how awful her life is with a non-speaking autistic child.

On the flip side, Tina, a parent carer to an autistic 10 year old, told me that she is often criticised for admitting online that she initially found her son's diagnosis overwhelming and terrifying. While they have now found their groove and Tina feels optimistic and confident about their lives together, she has often felt that not everyone wants to hear that acceptance of a long-term caring situation isn't always instant. Not everyone begins at the same point, and she believes we need to allow for people experiencing a diagnosis differently. To a proudly autistic adult, hearing of a parent's despair when their child receives a diagnosis can feel like a slap in the face. Despite the work of autistic advocates and charities, many people still think an autism diagnosis is almost as bad as a terminal one. But, as Tina says: 'It felt daunting because it was the unknown, not because I didn't love him, was ashamed or was trying to deny who he was. He was and will always be my son but I was frightened and sometimes still am.'

Sarah Roberts, too, has received criticism from other parents of children with Down's syndrome, for talking about some of the harder challenges. She told me she believes that at the root of it is a fear that if an expectant parent receives a prenatal diagnosis and comes across anything too negative, it will increase the likelihood they'll have an abortion. Sarah understands the feelings that drive those parents to criticise her, and she tries not to take it too personally. But it's not easy being told to be quiet by the same group of people you turn to for support. She has always strived for balance in how she presents her life, something she said is often missing from conversations about raising a child with Down's syndrome.

The online world can be a minefield for new carers to navigate. There is a proliferation, particularly by parent carers, of negative, ill-informed and dehumanising language about the disabled children they care for. In the world of autism, there is a camp of parent carers who speak about their children as if they aren't deserving of the same respect typical children are. War-like language such as warrior, battle and fight are used when talking about their children's disabilities. They write about how autism has negatively affected their own lives, how much they hate it, often blaming the child themselves, saying they are hard to love and need to be fixed. When this is the dominant tone of blogs that parents of newly diagnosed children are coming across, it's no wonder the wider autistic community bristles whenever a parent carer speaks about their experiences. But to dismiss the honest fears of parent carers is not the answer either.

In the months after my son's diagnosis I would lie awake at night feeling like I was floating away on a dark ocean. Our life had diverged from the course it had been set to and I was sailing far away from everything and everyone I knew. I didn't know where I was on a map. There were no recognisable landmarks. I had a strong feeling that we would find our way eventually but I could do almost nothing to control when that would happen. In the way that grief tends to behave, memories of my mother's death returned and I experienced those feelings like they were brand new. The old resentments that I had not felt for years resurfaced. Resentment that she had been too unwell to parent me through my teenage years in a way that I needed. Resentment that she was not here now when I needed her more than ever. I had almost forgotten those feelings. As if I had buried them long ago when we had buried her.

I didn't speak with anyone about the emotions that arose during that time. I could barely recognise myself in them. I would see a mother and son walking hand in hand down the street and I would feel a spike of jealousy in my chest so strong it felt like an electric shock. My son was nowhere near being able to walk calmly down a street holding my hand and he couldn't yet say a word. At seven months old, covered in spaghetti in her high chair, my daughter waved at me for the first time and, after the initial burst of joy, I felt an intense sadness; it took me a few moments to realise where it was coming from. Her older brother had never waved at me. It was the first of so many milestones that my daughter would reach before him. Rationally I knew it didn't matter. Rationally I knew he was on his own timeline. But it took time for my emotions to catch up with what I knew to be true.

I look back now at those early days of knowing my child had a lifelong disability and there is so much I wish I could give myself. There was almost no support available from the NHS due to underfunding of services, and we were pretty much sent on our way. There was no counselling, no guidance, no plan of action for how best we could support his needs, just a letter of diagnosis and a promise that we would get to attend a National Autistic Society parents' course at some point when we got to the top of the waiting list. It turned out to be about nine months later, by which time I had spent every evening researching it myself, alone in my kitchen. The result was we were left completely alone to figure out how to support Arthur's needs, with almost no guidance until he started school.

But more than professional advice, what I needed most was to see myself reflected in the world. When caring, disability and illness are hidden and never spoken about, we can feel we are the only ones struggling. We are in our own ocean, bobbing alone, not realising just how close we are to each other – so close that we could reach out and touch each other. Instead we stay in the dark for a long time, not talking about our experiences. What takes time to discover is that we are far from alone. We are in fact a large minority, distinct in that almost everyone will join our ranks at some point in their lives. When we do feel ready, when we open up, we see that all the ugly feelings, the jealousy, the sadness, the fear and the failure are not at all unique. Research Professor Brené Brown, who has spent two decades studying vulnerability, shame and empathy, describes shame as deriving its power from being unspeakable. Language and story, she says, bring light to shame and destroys it.[21] The stories of carers, just like the stories of those they care for, have long been shrouded in darkness. To speak up and share the conflicting feelings around caring is to peel away some of those shadows and form connections with others.

Whether or not you have supported a loved one with a disability or chronic illness, what follows in these pages are stories from those from whom we all have much to learn. As we navigate our roles as carers, these stories show that we are far from alone. Our situations might all be very different but we also have a huge amount in common. We must all somehow figure out the fine line of boundaries, confront our perfectionism, unpick our views on disability, build communities around us, learn to see the joys in a life we didn't necessarily choose, all while looking after our own health. It's certainly no easy task. We can't do it without the support of the wider community.

With all the best intentions in the world, whether we are daughters, parents, siblings or partners, we so often fall short. No one likes to admit they feel like they are failing at something so important. I sometimes fail to be the carer I want to be to my son. But when we speak up about the intricacies, the joys and the sorrows of our lives as carers, the fear and shame start to loosen their grip. When others hear our stories, they are able to step up and support us in the often intense job of caring for another human.

CHAPTER 2

Perfectionism

'The single greatest enemy of contemporary satisfaction may be the belief in human perfectibility.'[22]

Alain De Botton, philosopher and author

We had an awful night. I heard my son calling out to me, dragging me from a deep sleep. As soon as I'd registered the darkness and the feeling of too little sleep, my stomach felt heavy. I reached for my phone, sending off a silent prayer that it was later than I suspected. When the time 2.30am flashed up I was filled with dread. The school bus was more than five hours away. We had only had 4 hours' sleep and I could hear by the tone of his voice there would be no more sleep for us tonight. An hour later we are both sitting on the kitchen floor. I'm crying and Arthur is reciting scripts from favourite TV programmes to himself, a self-soothing technique he uses. A combination of thrown food, panic over blankets not being straight, and Arthur's refusal to let me go upstairs to see his sister when his shouts woke her have brought us here. I'm crying because I reacted in rage and shouted back. I'm crying because at times like these I wish I was a robot, with no feelings to get in the way. Or a cool and slightly emotionally distanced school teacher who never gets in a flap. To be the calm, indestructible foundation which my son can throw himself against. We hugged and I told him I was sorry and he used the only abstract language he knows: 'Sorry Mummy', which is heart-breaking. I was so tired and it dawned on me we were both probably coming down with the cold my daughter had. Arthur's already low tolerance for stress disappears when he is ill. My practised ability to cope with meltdowns also lowers dramatically. It feels so unfair that I'm not better at this for him. That on a night when he needs my steady presence I add fuel to his fires by reacting in exhaustion and anger. I know now after years of this that it will only make things worse if I beat myself up. But I still wish for the impossible. To be a perfect parent.

For a long time I didn't think I had particularly high expectations of myself as a parent to a disabled child. I was just doing what I thought was needed. In fact it felt like the bare minimum. I don't have high standards, I would tell myself. He deserves the best from me. But it was never enough. It never even felt close to being enough. Endless evenings were spent researching therapies and early interventions. Contrary to many people's assumptions, once Arthur was given a diagnosis we were pretty much waved on our way with no support. No person to turn to, no plan of action, barely any interventions. We were virtually on our own until he started school, and any support we received I had to find myself – with little guidance from anyone.

I spent hours poring over websites trying to figure out what to do next. I was overloading on articles and studies and private therapists extolling the necessity of early intervention. Fear-riddled articles about what must happen before they turn three, before five, definitely before the age of seven. Or it will *never* happen. Families telling the miraculous stories of the discovery of X therapy that transformed their child's life, after only two years full time and $200,000 in fees and lost income. 'But wouldn't you do *anything* to help your child?' it would read. Wouldn't any good parent quit their job/increase their mortgage/move across the country/insert massive life change here to ensure that their child had the best possible chance at gaining vital life skills? I faced a tsunami of information and a thousand ways to spend a lot of money or a lot of time, or both. Each story would be similar: 'We had almost given up hope, we had tried so many things, then X therapy came along and it changed our lives and now little Johnny walks, talks, eats, sleeps and shits just liked we dreamed he would. Don't give up hope! There is a therapy out there that will work for your child. Where there is a will there is a way! If you believe it enough, it will happen.' An horrific combination of ableism and consumerism at work to squeeze money out of fear-filled parents.

Perfectionism is a topic that came up again and again when I spoke to other parent carers. Perhaps the very high expectations put on parents generally in society right now make us vulnerable to it compared with caring situations involving other kinds of relationships. Although the pressure can be very high in all kinds of caring situations, the feeling that you are never doing a good enough job seems to overwhelm many parents, which is why parent carers are the main focus in this chapter.

When you are supporting a partner or parent, there may be times when they're able to assuage your fears somewhat, letting you know that what you are doing is enough. Of the disabled adults I spoke to, all of them expressed their gratitude for their relationships, for all the things their partner did to support them and for their good fortune at having a partner who both supported them and understood their need for as much independence as possible. No such reassurances exist as a parent, whether you are raising a disabled child or not. Perhaps it is also that constant background fear we have of who will look after our child after we are gone that has us mounting unsustainable pressure on ourselves. If we can just squeeze in more therapy, if we can just try a little harder, maybe that dark voice inside our heads will quieten down a little; the one that knows we have no answer to the question: what will happen to my child when I die?

When do I get to just be a mother?

Jess Moxham and I discussed those early days of seemingly insurmountable pressure, over cinnamon buns and coffee. Our boys were born within days of each other in hospitals only a couple of miles apart but their disabilities are quite different. Ben was born very ill and has cerebral palsy. He is a wheelchair user, has limited mobility in his hands and uses a feeding tube. Jess remembers the intense pressure of therapy in those first few years. One day, she recalls, she compiled a list of all the exercises from the occupational therapist, the speech therapist and the physiotherapist, along with all the medical appointments, tube feeding and nappy changing, and there were literally not enough hours in the day. 'When do I actually get to just be his mother?' she thought to herself.

Among the stories we both read online of other mothers doing extraordinary things for their children, she and I had similar reactions. Do we give up our jobs and be 100% focused on our child in order for them to meet their full potential? If I don't do that am I a bad mother? It always came down to the same thing in these stories. If you sacrificed enough, you would succeed. It felt to me as though anything less than perfect was not going to be good enough. And I felt like I was breaking apart under the pressure. Endless thoughts would run through my head. What would happen if music therapy was *the thing* for Arthur? If we don't try it we will never know. What if he gets to 18 and he still can't do XYZ and I will never know if it's because we didn't try music therapy? So we have to try music therapy. Can we afford it? Can we travel an hour each way for a 30-minute session? We have to do it or I will never know. But, of course, perfectionism always has another answer. If I try it and it's not helpful, it's probably because I didn't try hard enough.

Inherent in these perfectionist ideas is the pervasive ableism of our society. Our culture tells me both overtly and indirectly that if my son can't speak or interact easily it's because I'm not trying hard enough. Or perhaps that he's not trying hard enough. Either way, the idea of – as Alain De Botton puts it – 'human perfectibility' can only end in us all feeling like failures. When I see a parent sharing a hard moment online, expressing their sadness at not being able to hear their child's voice, it's often followed by comments telling them: 'Don't give up hope!' It makes me incredibly sad. We can have high hopes for our disabled children and yet still accept that verbal language may not be possible.

Jess tells me of a book she read about a child with cerebral palsy being taught to read and type by his mother after she quit her job and dedicated herself full time to the task. The school he had been attending didn't think it was achievable. Although the message of the book – the importance of presuming competence – was powerful, Jess found herself questioning her decisions about Ben after reading it. 'What if I'm the reason he can't read when he's older?' she says. I nod, recalling that familiar feeling of inadequacy which still creeps up on me. But we both agree it's crazy to think like that. Our boys each attend wonderful schools, with plenty of opportunities for learning and socialising and participating in life. And Jess, like myself, knows all too well the dangers of trying to be everything to our children. It can engulf you and your entire relationship if you take responsibility for all the therapy and learning, as well as the parenting. Jess had to quit her job as an architect long ago, not being able to enjoy the work when she couldn't commit to full-time hours. She is now a writer, which fits better with the needs of all three of her children. Even though we are both happier as working parents, reading stories of sacrifice by other mothers ending in incredible success leaves us both uneasy. What if what we are doing isn't enough?

Brené Brown explains in her work on perfectionism that in the West right now we are living in a culture of scarcity.[23] Scarcity can be described as 'never enough'. As a society, if we are constantly comparing and evaluating, we become hyperaware of what we lack. By comparing ourselves, our lives and our families to constructed images in the media, to a nostalgic idea of past or even to outliers, we will always find ourselves falling short. The opposite of scarcity is not abundance, it is simply enough. And it is an act of cultural defiance to even believe that we don't need to be constantly doing more in order to be seen as worthy.

Missing out on a magic ingredient

The thought of missing out on some magic ingredient of a therapy used to keep me awake at night. Arthur's development had begun fairly typically, aside from his early arrival into the world. In his first year I had trusted that he would show me what he needed. That he would interact and play and learn without too much thought on my part; just my presence, attention and love. As his second year passed I began to question my abilities as a mother. When he wasn't gloriously happy, he was utterly miserable. There seemed to be no in-between. He slept badly, pulled out his hair and started refusing much of the food he used to love. He went from exploring every piece of equipment in the playground to only wanting to be on a swing. I can now look back on those times and clearly see how his sensory difficulties were causing him so much distress. But at the time I could only think that I must have been missing some elusive piece of the puzzle that was motherhood.

It didn't help that other people noticed too. They were quick to point out all the things they were doing right that resulted in the perfect developmental specimen in their own pram. One mother at a baby group told me I should read to Arthur more if I wanted him to learn to speak. Another told me her child was so advanced because she 'just chatted to him all day long. You should do that.' I thought I was going crazy. But I *am* talking to him and reading to him and singing to him and playing with him, I would think. Am I doing it all wrong? It was as if all the mothers I knew had been given a spell, whispered into their ears at the birth of their child. The magic ingredient that someone had forgotten to tell me. Without that vital message I was not able to help Arthur. We were lost.

When he was a toddler and my friends were taking their children to baby gym classes and library reading sessions, I was taking online courses trying to learn how to stop him from attacking his baby sister. I didn't tell anybody. He was still undiagnosed but showing more and more signs of anxiety and a poor ability to cope with any kind of stress, and I found myself retreating from local friends. A day alone, in our own little bubble, seemed much safer than seeing him side by side with peers. As his differences became pronounced, particularly as his behaviour became aggressive, I found it upsetting to be around other children his age. I watched other parents, I examined how they interacted with their children and I tried to figure out what I was doing so wrong. I looked through books and threw each of them aside. None of them seemed to be speaking to my situation at all. I tried the 'love bombing' technique, a showering of love and undivided attention, but Arthur appeared to have a well in him so deep that my love never filled it. He rarely seemed satisfied and was often distressed.

One day when our kids were around two, a local mum friend and I were in the park, both of us also with newborns in slings. Arthur lashed out unexpectedly at my friend's daughter, who started crying hysterically. Embarrassed, I apologised, explaining that we were having a bit of an issue with hitting lately. She comforted her daughter and smiled at me, telling me not to worry. She went on to say that her daughter was just shocked because no one had ever hurt her before. 'She's never seen anyone hit before. She doesn't know what it is!' she said. My face glowed red and I felt sick to my stomach. I strapped Arthur into to his pushchair, mumbling something about him probably being tired, and I got away as soon as I could. I cried all the way home. Her child had never seen anyone hit and my child was lashing out at his baby sister and me daily. Had she thought Arthur had *learned* hitting at home? That her child was innocent and Arthur was not? What I read into her words was that I was alone and probably doing something to cause it.

Feelings of shame

I would look back at this incident over the coming years and see it for what it really was. It was the first time I had consciously experienced a deep sense of shame as a mother. The red-hot cheeks and overturned stomach would become a familiar physical manifestation of this shame, repeated again and again as I failed to live up to what I thought a mother should be. I wasn't ashamed of my son. I was ashamed of myself and all the things

I seemed to be missing that would support him better. The talk around café tables as our children grew older was of how much easier everything was getting, and all I could think was how nothing felt further from the truth. That I seemed to be in a topsy-turvy world where my son's needs only got more difficult to meet. From the blank expressions that confronted me when I revealed a snippet of what was happening, I figured they assumed I was doing something wrong. I have never felt more lonely in my life than when I thought everyone else knew how to be a good enough parent, and I did not.

The hitting became so distressing that I decided to take some action; I found an online course run by child psychologists that aimed to help your child stop hitting. Even though it was helpful, as I went through the course I had a growing sense of unease, which took me a while to pinpoint. The examples used by the therapist were all examples from her practice, with names changed to protect identities. They were all children who had experienced early childhood trauma. After one session I closed my laptop down and sobbed for half an hour as I realised the behaviour I was seeing in my son was almost identical to that of a young boy whose mother had left him alone every night as a baby to do a night shift as she had no one else to take care of him. Although it was only a few months later that we began to pursue an autism diagnosis, the feeling of potentially being the cause of my son's extreme distress did not disappear overnight. While I may not have blamed myself for the actual diagnosis, I piled a mounting pressure on myself to help support his needs as best I could. With little guidance from anyone and no idea what 'good enough' even looked like, it was an endless pursuit with no answer and no end.

Sarah Roberts, whose eldest son Oscar has Down's syndrome (see Chapter 1, page 26), says that she sometimes feels as if she can never get it right. At parties and gatherings, she always has half her attention on what Oscar is up to, only half listening to what anyone else is saying. She's often accused of being a 'helicopter parent' but if she doesn't stick close enough to him and something happens, she's seen as irresponsible. While this is a common feeling among modern mothers – that they are damned if they do and damned if they don't – it's taken to a whole other level when you are the parent to a disabled child. Perhaps sometimes a parent might be projecting the idea of being judged on to a situation when no one is even really paying attention to us. But not always. Sarah feels there is a high expectation about Oscar's behaviour, and occasionally criticism for her when he doesn't meet those expectations. It adds unnecessary pressure.

These days a difficult morning can begin with one innocuous, badly phrased comment. Arthur's school bus comes to our door, and if he's upset they refuse to take him, so I carefully manage our mornings to make them as smooth as possible. But a poorly timed grumpy word from me, or a prompt to eat a bit faster, may be all it takes to have everything turned upside down, the school bus driving away without him. This leads to the logistical night-mare of getting two kids to two different schools for the same start time, a change in routine which leaves Arthur even more upset and creates emotional exhaustion all round. It's hard not to berate myself over mistakes that can send both our mornings off in a disastrous direction.

These incidents, and the fear of them, have me trying to control everything I possibly can. But it's an impossible task. Sometimes we have only slept for three hours. Other times my mind is occupied with worries about money and overdue invoices, or the babysitter calling in sick, or my daughter's asthma flaring up, and I just don't have the capacity to get it right every time.

Other times I make mistakes like mentioning the beach holiday that is still two days from now, and realise too late that I'm now in for hours of repeated asking to go to the beach – a loop Arthur gets stuck in of either something he desperately wants or something he desperately wants to avoid. I silently beat myself up as I hear him ask to go in the car for the hundredth time in 30 minutes, as he gets more and more distressed. That elusive grip over the concept of time that has him struggle with anything beyond what's happening next. And I know it's my fault as he spirals into anxiety about when exactly we are going to the beach. Two days from now might as well be two centuries.

One day I accidentally knocked a glass of water onto Arthur's duvet which he had dragged into the kitchen to play on. At bed time when it was still not dry, I managed to convince him to use our spare one. After an extended and restless bedtime, it worked and he fell asleep, curled up entirely under it, as he always does. But my relief at having figured out a solution didn't last long, as he was awake and dripping with sweat by 1am. I had forgotten the spare duvet was a thick winter one and Arthur can't sleep without something entirely covering him. Not a big deal, perhaps, except that he can never fall asleep again after waking in the night and it was the third 1am start I had had with him in a week. I dragged myself through the following day and all I could think about was how bloody stupid I was to knock that glass of water over.

Throwaway comments, spilt water, running out of the right kind of snack, timing a car trip incorrectly: these may be tiny annoyances to many, but to my son they can be a source of extreme distress. As a parent I tread the line carefully between preparing him for the imperfect stuff of life which we must all learn to tolerate, and keeping his mind as calm as possible in order to learn and interact with a world he finds overwhelming and very difficult to process. I try to control the world around him to make it easier for him to be in. But it's impossible and I fail often.

Letting go of control

Lois Prislovsky is an educational psychologist who became the long-time collaborator, co-author and friend to non-speaking autistic Barb Rentenbach. Barb and Lois have written two books together, sharing Barb's experiences as an autistic woman, about the power of connection and the friendship that formed between them. Lois says that the strong desire to control outcomes for our children and loved ones needs to be let go if the whole family is going to thrive. She has worked with countless families of neuro-divergent children over the years, and thinks that the need to control only leads to anxiety, and it's too high a price to pay. Her advice to me, as she spoke over Skype from her home in California, is to forget outcomes and accept you cannot be everything to your child – although she admits it is a lot harder than it sounds. You cannot control outcomes even for yourself, let alone another human. If we can live in the now, enjoy our kids, do what we can and accept that whatever happens will be for the best, she says we will have the best chance of a good outcome anyway. 'Release control of what is not yours to control.' It takes practice, Lois says, but the alternative is a life of high anxiety, and that's no good for anyone. She laughs at the idea anyone could control Barb. 'Barb is uncontrollable! But in the most powerful way.' I laugh too, because I could say exactly the same for Arthur, who knows his own mind better than any child I've ever met and will not be swayed by anyone or anything. Not that I haven't tried.

How does letting go of control and of outcomes help us live more fulfilled lives as carers? Brené Brown describes perfectionism as 'the belief that if we live perfect, look perfect, and act perfect, we can minimise or avoid the pain of blame, judgment and shame.'[24] She says it's a twenty-tonne shield that we think will protect us but in fact is the very thing that holds us back. It's not difficult for me to look back at all the times that I have thought to myself that *if I can just get this right* then I know I will have done everything I can to support Arthur. Except I can never get it right. Arthur is not a doll or a pet to control and manipulate. He has his own very strong thoughts and feelings about what he will and will not do, as well as his own intense challenges which I may never fully understand. The more I allow perfectionist thinking to rule me, the more likely I am to fall apart when I inevitably fail. The more likely I am to give up. And, more worryingly, that Arthur will learn to feel as though nothing he does is good enough either.

It has taken me a long while to see that my fear of judgment and blame from society – for not being able to help Arthur to speak, behave and learn as his peers do – is hiding an ugly truth. That once upon a time I would judge and blame others for their own difficulties. I would question whether what they were doing was enough. Are they really trying hard enough? Are they doing everything they can to help themselves? Where does this blame and judgment come from? It's from that deep fear inside that we are *all* vulnerable to not being able to control our lives and some of the things that happen to us. That we may be utterly vulnerable in this world and there is no medicine or therapy or treatment or intervention that can change that. It is easier to blame and shame others than it is to admit there are things in this world that are beyond our control. It can feel terrifying to let go.

Tanya Savva was already working as an occupational therapist when her daughter Mackenzie was born. It was discovered not long after her birth, when she wasn't feeding well or growing, that she had a mid-brain malformation which caused a number of issues, including blindness and no pituitary gland function. When Mackenzie was seven weeks old, Tanya was told that she would probably never eat orally, walk or talk. Tanya, like Jess Moxham, describes the first couple of years as firefighting and just keeping Mackenzie alive. Feeding was a huge problem for her, so an NG tube was inserted (a feeding tube that goes in through the nostril and down into the stomach) which at eight months was switched to a peg (a device inserted into the stomach so that formula can be inserted directly, bypassing the mouth altogether). This was followed by two-and-a-half years of chronic vomiting so, despite the peg, Mackenzie still struggled to put on weight. Finally, Tanya went against her doctor's advice and ditched the formula and started putting puréed food into her daughter's tube. It worked almost instantly. The vomiting stopped and Mackenzie started to thrive.

Tanya, with her experience and understanding of the body and typical development from her job as an OT, was able to strongly advocate for her daughter and apply everything she was being recommended by physios and feeding therapists to a very high standard. They did intensive amounts of feeding therapy to combat her oral aversion and Mackenzie slowly learned to eat. The physio was also successful and Mackenzie started weight bearing and walking. But this came with a downside. 'The OT hat never came off,' Tanya told me. After years of intervening with her daughter's therapy, Tanya got to the point that she realised they never simply played. Every activity had a purpose and therapeutic function. 'By the time she was five, I was so over being her therapist, I wanted to be her mum.' Between her work as an OT and all the therapy she was doing to support Mackenzie, Tanya felt she was burning the candle at both ends, and finally realised it was unsustainable.

The necessity and burden of therapy

The difficulty is that taking your child to therapy once a week or once a fortnight is simply not enough. It is essential for us as carers to follow through with interventions that the medical professionals teach us. We are well placed to do so as loving and present family members, and we do have a responsibility to do so. But along with that, Tanya explains, we also need to come to terms with the fact it might not always be possible, and that brings with it huge amounts of guilt and shame. Feeling either like we haven't done enough to help our kids thrive, or never feeling we get to just be 'mum'.

In the end, Tanya took a drastic measure to change both her and Mackenzie's life. She quit her job as a full-time occupational therapist in Sydney, bought a caravan, took Mackenzie out of school and hit the road, travelling up the coast of Australia for six months. Within a few weeks, she realised that the list of interventions she had intended to practise with her daughter wasn't going to happen. She couldn't do it all and something had to give. Tanya says she made the decision to surrender to the trip and wait and see what happened. Despite the constant travel – which can be challenging for anyone with both sensory issues and visual impairment – the caravan became a safe base through which to explore the world. Everything was set up in a way to enable Mackenzie to be as independent as possible, and their slow pace of life on the road had her cooking, being in nature, swimming and walking in challenging environments like rainforests and beaches. So while the traditional therapies were abandoned, Mackenzie's development came on in leaps and bounds as she explored the country with her mother.

The closeness of the caravan meant that Tanya also had a new appreciation for just how extreme Mackenzie's anxiety was.

Lying next to her each night, she would hear her calm, long sleeping breaths become short and held even before she opened her eyes each morning. Tanya hadn't quite realised the extent to which her daughter was in a constant state of high alert at every waking moment. Back in Sydney, between full-time work, school and therapy, there had been hardly any time in the day among all the rushing to realise how intense things were for Mackenzie. The slow pace of the road meant Tanya could really appreciate just how Mackenzie's anxiety affected the way she interacted with the world.

After they returned to Sydney, Tanya decided to go back to studying. The trip had made her realise she had no interest in returning to her old ways of intense, long days. She took her skills with the human body and retrained as a yoga teacher and massage therapist, completing training to become a coach. After another summer on the road in the caravan with Mackenzie, she had the idea of creating retreats for mothers of disabled kids, to give them the space and opportunity to relax and recharge in a supportive environment. It is this work with other mothers that helped Tanya see the immense pressure we put ourselves under when it comes to our disabled children. If parenting naturally comes with its fair share of guilt, then parenting a disabled child takes it to another level. While escaping the pressures of city life for a time was an effective way to step off the therapy/school/work treadmill for Tanya, most of us won't be able to take such a drastic step. But I think we *can* all learn to slow down and take stock of what's really important, without abandoning our homes and lives in the process.

External pressures

Along with internal pressures, there are also intense pressures from the outside to be the 'perfect' carer. In almost every initial meeting I have with a professional in relation to Arthur, I'm expected to lay out all the ways in which I am already trying to support his needs myself before I can access additional help. My parenting is scrutinised in a way none of my friends raising non-disabled kids experience. As his mother and main carer, I'm expected to be impeccable in every way before more money is spent. I find myself defensive and justifying my pleas for help whenever I'm up against a gatekeeper. And it does feel like I am up against them. Meetings are generally spent reminding me just how many children their services need to provide for. Just how many people are in a worse situation than our family. It's hard not to let the shame creep in or to think I should be able to handle this all myself without help.

This is a feeling shared by most parent carers I have spoken to. Claire Kotecha's 10-year-old son Anand has a rare cerebral palsy that means he requires support for every aspect of his care. He has recently begun to require not just one-to-one support but one-to-one nursing care. Claire can no longer take her eyes off him for a moment in case he aspirates (when saliva makes its way into his windpipe and he can't breathe). This means someone needs to be awake to watch Anand while he's sleeping, someone needs to be sitting beside him on every car journey, and with him every moment of the day. Claire, like so many other carers, has had to go to a panel to get extra support now that his needs go beyond what she can physically cope with. At first she was told that she should be the one staying awake all night with him and that she could sleep for the six hours he attended school each day. Never mind that Claire has another child, has her own needs to meet, has mountains of medical paperwork, and the up to 150 medical and therapy appointments she needs to get Anand to each year. When the default position of the Local Authority, medical staff and teachers is that we are not doing enough, it can be impossible not to berate ourselves when we cannot meet those expectations.

Claire argued her point and was given night support. Anand now has a nurse arriving at 10pm each night so that Claire and her husband Dipen can get enough sleep in order to be there for Anand the rest of the day. Claire is now on a quest to try and get an evening of nursing once every couple of weeks, so that she and Dipen can have an evening out together. She's already been told no once, but she's not giving up. Apparently, as a two-parent family, social services feel there is no reason why they need that support. Having time together as a couple every now and again is not a need they see as important. Not long after we spoke, Claire and Dipen were given an extra 2.5 hours a month to spend an evening together.

I asked Claire how confident she feels about meeting Anand's needs since his breathing worsened. She sighed and said that a year ago when things changed, they both took training in how to use suction to clear his airways. After the first training they tried to make her sign a waiver form, saying she was competent to do it. She refused, terrified she wouldn't be able to do it properly or that she would injure him. She made them train her two more times before she reluctantly signed. In the end, Claire explains, she hated the idea that she would have to rely on someone else to keep Anand safe. She wants to be the one doing it. It's hard enough that she now needs a nurse with her when she drives Anand to his medical appointments, or out and about with their younger daughter. She would much rather be able to meet all Anand's needs herself because she's happy to do it. But there is only so much one person can do. She's been told by social workers that they already have more than most people and should be

grateful, rather than asking for more. With social services funding stressed beyond capacity, it's widely agreed that there is a
crisis in social care.[25] But reminding carers that there are others
who have needs, as if what we ask for is unreasonable, is not a
fair response to a parent simply trying to meet their child's needs.
Claire is grateful. Incredibly so. And unwavering in her belief
that she's doing the best one person can despite a system not set
up to support her son's high needs.

Claire's readiness to fight for Anand's needs, and her own as
his main carer, is a reminder of the ways in which the medical
and educational systems set us up to question ourselves and our
abilities as carers. Though it may not be their intention, we are
sometimes treated as though we could be doing more and doing
it better. We are treated this way largely because there is not
enough money to go around and anyone seen to be coping
is dismissed. If we haven't driven ourselves to the brink of a
breakdown, we have not done enough to deserve help. The short-
sightedness of this way of thinking is staggering, and dangerous
to the disabled children and adults reliant on us being fit and
well. It can take a huge amount of confidence to stand up for
yourself and say, 'I am doing enough,' when everyone else expects
more and more of you. Some carers I have spoken to have been
treated as selfish or greedy for asking for more help in what are
quite dire circumstances.

How can we not be perfectionists when we are prodded for
proof of our efforts from every professional who crosses our
path? Funding is so tight that carers are expected to move
heaven and earth for a paltry £66-a-week Carer's Allowance.
Within social services and the NHS, individuals with extraordinary kindness exist, but it's a broken system. I meet kind
and sympathetic people saying that they wish they didn't have
to ask these questions and they wish there was more they

could do. I come away from appointments drained from arguing our case, in tears over being questioned about how much more I could be doing. Undone by the endless feeling of 'never enough'.

Rebecca (not her real name), whose 17-year-old daughter has struggled with addiction and mental illness for years, told me that in the area of child mental health she is often overtly blamed for her daughter's difficulties. Her daughter has been sectioned twice and each time her file states 'permissive parenting' as one of her problems. Rebecca said that she is mentioned countless times in her daughter's files. As a mother she is treated as the cause of the problem, despite the fact she has been asking for help for many years. Pleas which were ignored until her daughter took an overdose. Very recently, after years of struggling to get support, her daughter finally received a formal diagnosis of ADHD and PTSD, the latter brought on by a sexual assault. Rebecca is furious that it took so long for her daughter's needs to be recognised and that she had been blamed all these years for being a bad parent. She finally feels they are now on the right path, starting to access the right help.

Carers need compassion

If we are to live in a world where we can look ourselves in the mirror and say 'I did enough today', then we need compassion *from* a system that expects too much from us. In one day I can go from a dentist telling me I'm feeding my son too much fruit (after being praised for managing the same by the paediatrician a week earlier), and a therapist questioning my coping skills after I asked for more support, to a new teacher assuming, from my son's challenging behaviours, that there are no boundaries at home. Perfectionist fires are stoked by flames of austerity, budget cuts and a government getting by on supporting disabled people with the bare minimum.

We may not have control over how we are treated, and we may be expected to perform above and beyond what many would deem acceptable, but we do have some control over ourselves: over those moments in the mirror when we must defy the messages we receive daily and instead say to ourselves, 'I am doing enough. I'm not perfect, but I'm enough.' It is hard. Brené Brown calls it a constant and daily act of defiance against society. 'The larger culture is always applying pressure, and unless we are willing to push back and fight for what we believe in, the default becomes a state of scarcity.'[26]

I continue to practise. Some days it feels easier. Some days it feels impossible. And because of this, learning to have compassion for ourselves is essential, something I explore more in a later chapter. Without extending compassion to myself I cannot experience it for all those other carers who have been filling out paperwork, fielding phone calls, worrying about bills and having sleepless nights. And, perhaps more importantly, nor can I extend it to my son.

In clinging to ideas of perfectibility, what am I teaching him, a child who struggles to do things that others find easy? By applying pressure to myself to find answers that may unlock his potential, I am inadvertently telling him he is not enough just as he is. Sally Derby (see Chapter 1, page 27) pointed out to me when we spoke that, as a disabled woman, she doesn't need perfection from her husband (who provides support for her), she just needs some understanding. For her that means he gets that she wants to be as independent as possible but that he also recognises that she sometimes struggles to ask for help.

It is entirely possible to be both full of hope for Arthur's future and not – as Lois Prislovsky points out – fixated on certain outcomes. His future will be different to how I imagined it was going to be back when he was a chubby six-month-old baby meeting all his milestones. Accepting difference does not mean giving up hope. Accepting that I will never be a perfect parent or carer does not mean giving up on being a good parent. It means accepting my own limitations with kindness. The sort of kindness I hope my son gives himself when he struggles to achieve something his peers find relatively simple.

Jess Moxham told me about the day things began to change for her. Her husband James, who works long hours during the week, was curled up on the sofa with Ben one weekend, the two of them watching the rugby together. Jess felt annoyed that they were 'just sitting there' and started questioning why he wasn't doing physio with Ben. James turned around to look at her and said, 'I just want to hang out with my son and watch the rugby.' It was the moment, Jess says, that she started to shift her thinking from trying to do as much as possible for Ben, to allowing him to be a little boy. Slowing down the constant striving was a process, but over time she realised Ben would be ok with a little less therapy. And the whole family would benefit from just relaxing and spending time together. Just as Arthur will be ok if I don't try every intervention. We will all be ok, if we can look at ourselves and remember that we are enough, just as we are.

CHAPTER 3

Ableism

'Know that freaking out is ok. Now know that a lot of what you're freaking out about is misinformation, so you can stop freaking out.'[27]

Jess Wilson, writer and parent advocate

'I am disguised as a poor thinker.'[28]

Barb Rentenbach, author and non-speaking autistic

Ableism Definition: The discrimination against and prejudice towards disabled people

In the days after giving birth to her daughter at 32 weeks, Alice Bennett made the first of many decisions to advocate for her daughter. She had known from around 17 weeks into her pregnancy that Raya had hydrocephalus, a neural tube defect which meant that the fluid that is produced by the brain cannot be drained properly, causing dangerous swelling. The neurosurgeon who stood in front of her explaining the life-saving surgery her baby would need was the same surgeon who had, in every one of the many prenatal appointments, told her that her child would have no quality of life and be a burden on her. She had been offered and even pressured to have an abortion throughout, despite telling her medical team over and over that she had made her decision and wanted them to stop asking her. Alice was incredulous. So much so that after Raya's birth she made the decision to refuse to let her be treated by that surgeon and demanded a different one. She felt unable to trust this man with her daughter's life, when he had made it clear that he thought that Alice would be better off without her. Under a new surgeon, Raya's first two surgeries were a success and they were allowed to go home after four weeks. Alice had learned very early that she was raising her daughter in a world where not everyone believed she deserved the same chances as everyone else. Even the medical professionals she was supposed to trust. She was just 17 years old.

Disability has long been hidden from the mainstream, and for many people becoming a carer may be their first experience of it. We rarely see disabled people on TV, in films or in books. The stories being told aren't written by disabled people, so when we do see disabled characters, it's often from a non-disabled point of view. Few of our policy makers or leaders are disabled, which is reflected in the poor funding of social care services, specialist education and NHS services for those with chronic illnesses and lifelong disabilities. Encountering ableism up close and personal for the first time when we see the way a loved one is spoken to, treated, dismissed, devalued or ignored, can be a very rude awakening. But none of this is news to disabled people. They have been experiencing it all of their lives.

What is easy to forget, though, is that despite not being aware of it, despite it being hidden from our eyes, we are all shaped by the ableist culture in which we live. And it is this shaping that is the cause of so much unnecessary sorrow when someone we love becomes, or is born, disabled and we are thrown unexpectedly into the role of carer. Understanding disability discrimination and how society views disabled people can be the key to understanding why we might have so many difficult feelings about someone we love being disabled or chronically ill.

The Equality Act 2010 (UK) defines disability as a mental or physical condition or impairment that has a substantial and long-term negative effect on your ability to do normal everyday activities.[29]

In all my conversations with other carers one thing is universal. Every one of them has been told that they are exceptional for loving and supporting a disabled family member. When an acquaintance gives me a misty-eyed look and a tilted head when I talk about what to me is our ordinary lives, a deeply uncomfortable feeling of distance comes between us. When people make carers out to be exceptional, they are implying (whether consciously or not) that the person we support is hard to love. When they sigh and say, 'I don't know how you do it,' what they're really saying is, 'thank god that's not me.'

This is why the conversation around ableism and the rights of disabled people is vital for carers too. How can we come to terms with our role supporting a partner, child or parent if every message we receive in films, literature, advertising, politics – whether through omission or negative single narratives – is that disability is among the worst things that could happen to you?

First encounters with disability

I vividly remember my first known encounter with an autistic person. I was an obsessive reader as a child and almost nothing brought me more joy than the arrival of the latest *Baby-Sitters Club* book. In one particular book, Kirsty, club president, begins to look after an eight-year-old girl Susan, who is autistic and has largely been hidden away by her family. Through the book Kirsty struggles to connect with the girl – who has savant syndrome, is exceptional at the piano and is non-speaking. Although in the end the author tries to sell the message that 'we are all different and that's ok', that wasn't the impression I was left with. What I remember was how ashamed the family were of their daughter, how they kept her secret from the neighbourhood and how they hoped their next baby would give them a chance at a 'normal family'. Thirty years after I read the book I can still remember a scene where Kirsty drags a screaming Susan away from her piano because she thinks it would be good for her to play outside. I put the book down, and despite the attempt at an uplifting ending, all I could think was that having an autistic child must be the worst thing that could happen to you.

Although I have since had many encounters with autistic people, it undoubtedly shaped my impressions. There are cultural touch points that get stored away in our minds that, as Laura Dorwart (see Chapter 1, page 31) says, make up a constellation of impressions of a particular disability.[30] But what happens when those impressions are made and controlled largely by non-disabled people? The author of *The Baby-Sitters Club*, as far as I'm aware, was not autistic but had spent a short amount of time looking after an autistic child. When the stories of disabled people are told through the lens of a non-disabled person, we get a very narrow view of disability. Narrow, misrepresented and often negative. A singular narrative of hardship, something broken to be fixed or eradicated. Or perhaps the flip side of that: a story of overcoming that hardship in order to be an inspiration. What we know about a particular disability is made up of a few whispered conversations, a TV movie and a badly formed character in a children's book series.

For Hayley Newman, when her daughter Natty's Down's syndrome was identified immediately after birth, her first impressions of Down's sprung to mind. She was four or five years old and walking down the street, holding her grandmother's hand. Ahead of them was a man with Down's syndrome and a woman, probably his mother. Hayley's grandmother steered them very deliberately across the street to avoid them. Hayley watched them walk by, their heads lowered to avoid eye contact, at the embarrassment at having been so obviously avoided. Hayley's grandmother bent down to her and whispered, 'he's not all there,' and carried on walking. Her much beloved grand-mother had inadvertently shaped Hayley's first thoughts and fears as she watched over her baby daughter in the neonatal intensive care unit. Someone people cross the street to avoid. While her grandmother's opinions may have come from another generation, views such as these trickle down and still affect the lives of people living today.

The day we first discussed the possibility of an autism diagno-sis for Arthur was not a particularly sad day for me. I had already been turning it over in my mind for months, and that was after more months of being too terrified to type anything into Google in case my suspicions were confirmed. By the time the long-awaited appointment arrived I was fairly certain that though Arthur's development was delayed, he was also developing differently.

Although the word autism didn't terrify me, something else was lurking beneath the surface which I couldn't voice and didn't dare think about. The idea that he might be an autistic child who remained non-speaking, visibly and obviously disabled, having to attend a special school outside of our neighbourhood, segre-gated and excluded from mainstream life. Autism I can handle, I thought to myself. Non-speaking, intellectually disabled and autistic? I couldn't even say those words in my head. The feelings of dread that crept up on me when I allowed even a glimmer of that future to come into my mind were utterly overwhelming. *It's not going to happen*, I repeated over and over to myself. What I would come to learn over the next few years was that the assumptions I made about life for autistic people had almost entirely been formed by non-autistic people's views about what did and did not constitute a good, valuable and worthwhile life. This is not specific to autism. How much do any of us really know about what it is like to live with a disability like multiple sclerosis, a spinal injury or visual impairment? Probably very little in reality and, as such, those words can appear utterly terrifying.

While I would hope that most people these days would agree that direct discrimination of disabled people is wrong, and that access – such as ramps – should be a human right, ableism runs far deeper than that in our culture. In her 1991 book *Pride Against Prejudice*, Jenny Morris explains that like the feminist movement, disability rights can be best understood through the 'personal as political' paradigm. Disabled people are not simply an 'add on' any more than women are an 'add on' to men. We don't turn to men to understand the experiences of women. Women need to tell their own stories in order for their rights and needs to be met. The disability movement, she argues, needs to be understood in the same way. Until disabled people's experiences are listened to and understood, their lives will be undervalued. She writes: 'Assumptions that our lives are not worth living are only possible when our subjective realities find no place in mainstream culture. Where disability is represented in the general culture it is primarily from the point of view of the non-disabled and so their fears and hostility, and their own cultural agendas, dominate the way we are presented.'[31]

Ableism is so deeply embedded in our culture that a non-disabled paediatric surgeon feels it's appropriate to give a new mother his personal opinion as to what does and does not constitute quality of life. While it is generally accepted that it is not morally right to make assumptions about a person based on their race, the same view is often not extended to disabled people. Morris argues that no person, other than the person concerned, has the right to claim what is and is not a life worth living. But with disability so feared and misunderstood by non-disabled people, when the only stories being told are through the lens of a non-disabled person, it will just perpetuate fear and misunderstanding.

In those dark days after my son's initial diagnosis I was gripped with fear. Fear that I had a child who was now bottom of the world pecking order, vulnerable to bullying and abuse, vulnerable to not having his educational needs met, vulnerable to ridicule and pity. Why were those my fears? Because everything about our culture tells me that is so. It's in the casual use of ableist slurs like retard and idiot. The almost complete invisibility of intellectually disabled adults in the world. It is our cultural obsession with productivity, with value attached to net worth, to fitting in rather than standing out. It is in the awkward words 'how awful' uttered by friends and acquaintances who don't know what else to say, when what we need to hear is, 'you're doing a really good job.' It's in the lack of invitations to attend birthday parties and the friendships that slowly fall by the wayside.

As a parent with a newly diagnosed child, or someone facing a new and life-changing diagnosis of a loved one, is it any wonder many experience feelings of deep sadness? Morris writes that disabled people face undermining messages each day about their value in the world. Those of us supporting disabled people have been exposed to those same messages. But whether or not we cling to that narrative is a choice.

Aly Grace is an autistic Australian writer who is also raising an autistic child. She writes that 'feelings about disabled children do not exist within a vacuum, but from within an ablest society that devalues them from birth and teaches others to do the same.'[32] As parents, partners, siblings and friends, one of the most important things we can do is begin to unpick and analyse all that we have been told about disability. Is it truth? Or is it a non-disabled point of view? The most effective way to do that is to not only question all that we see and are told but to seek out the voices of disabled people who are telling their own stories.

A different perspective

As I fumbled around online, trying to make sense of our new reality, I was overwhelmed by the kinds of information non-autistic people – mainly parents and medical professionals – were putting online. Diets, cures and anti-vax groups. Americans with health insurance paying for 50 hours a week of intensive therapy for their two and three year olds. Fifty hours a week! Most people I knew didn't work that many hours in their full-time jobs. It all felt so off. But what did I know? I didn't know anything much about autism. All the information I was coming across was from a perspective of deficits. But I was never going to get past my fears for both our futures so long as I was surrounded by people who considered my son lacking and a person to be trained and fixed. I knew I needed to find another way, or we'd both be miserable.

For me that began when I came across Jess Wilson's blog 'Diary of a Mom'. Jess's second daughter Brooke (not her real name) was diagnosed as autistic aged three, and Jess began writing her blog as a way of trying to make sense of their journey together. Over the years something changed for Jess. She went from feeling devastated and fearful to feeling optimistic and grateful. What changed? She discovered autistic adults, who wrote and talked about their own lived experiences. What she had thought was truth – that being autistic is a tragedy – was not in fact the truth at all.

Jess admits that the first time she heard the word autism in relation to her daughter, she retched over a toilet bowl. It took time for her to see that this bodily reaction was the direct result of the way disability, and autism in particular, is spoken about in our society. Large charities like Autism Speaks still depend on fear-mongering to raise money. When organisations rely on negative emotions – pity, sadness, fear – to fundraise, they are directly impacting the lives of those who are living with the disabilities, by shaping the opinions of people whose only knowledge of a certain disability might be through one of those charities. When Jess realised her fears were an internalisation of society's views of disability and were not always based on actual lived experience, things changed. She told me that she 'began to peel away the layers and started to be able to say ok, this is a multi-dimensional thing just like any other part of humanity. Parts of it are going to be hard, parts of it are going to suck and parts of it are going to unbelievably amazing.'

It was through Jess Wilson that I discovered the work of Barb Rentenbach. Barb, now in her mid-forties, is autistic, non-speaking and describes herself as 'disguised as a poor thinker.'[33] Barb's mother Barbara, whom Barb jokingly refers to as Smother, is a vivacious and energy-filled parent who was determined to give Barb as many opportunities as possible in life. When Barb was 19 she began the difficult task of learning to communicate through typing, or facilitated communication as it is often called. Barb wasn't particularly interested at first. It seemed like a lot of hard work and she had pretty much resigned herself to a life of pleasure and comfort, being fully cared for and not challenging herself too much. But she was surprised by how much she enjoyed the company of the young educational psychologist Lois Prislovsky, and soon realised she had an awful lot to say and contribute to the world from her unique perspective. They worked steadily at it and became friends and colleagues, eventually completing a book together over ten years. *I Might Be You* is about Barb's experiences as a non-speaking autistic woman and the connection that formed between her and Lois as they discovered a way for her to communicate with the world. The next book, *Neurodiversity*, a series of essays written alternately between Lois (who has ADHD) and Barb, took a much speedier four years to complete, and looks at how different people think and why we all need to lean in to our strengths.

When I spoke to Lois about their time together, she said that the most important thing to remember when working with people who are 'disguised as poor thinkers' is to treat them like brilliant thinkers. That means listening. Barb, who was finally able to communicate her interests more clearly through typing, wanted to read (and listen via audio books) about philosophy and history, focusing on the writing of neurodivergent thinkers. This was far more intellectually challenging than anyone had previously thought Barb capable of. Barb herself writes about how her own high school special education was so boring she mostly checked out mentally and spent time in her own mind. As soon as someone started to treat her as a person who might have intellectual interests, she began to thrive.

Reading Barb's words has allowed me a glimpse into a world I have never experienced myself. While no two people's experiences are ever going to be the same, her work has given me more insight into my son's life than I could possibly get from any non-autistic professional or expert. What it's like to struggle to communicate. What it's like to be treated as a 'poor thinker'. What it's like to be able to enjoy the world from an entirely different and all-encompassing sensory perspective. How wonderful, pleasure-filled and complete life can be, even without verbal language. Despite requiring personal care support around the clock for the most basic functions, Barb lives an incredibly rich and varied life. I look at Barb's life and I am not afraid for my son's future. All he and I need is the right support and he will have a life anyone would be proud of. Not an easy life. Barb is the first to admit being in an autistic body is anything but easy. But it is an excellent life.

If I look at these two examples of writing about non-speaking autistic people, *The Baby-Sitters Club*, versus Barb Rentenbach's two books, the difference is clear. One is the view from the outside in, from a non-disabled person's view of profound disability; a picture of difficulty, deficits and 'wrongness'. Perhaps it's unfair to look at a children's book from the 1980s. We could instead use the countless examples of contemporary autism memoirs written by non-disabled parents who give a very similar view. On the other hand, Barb's work from her own perspective, whilst not shying away from some of the intense difficulties she faces, is joyous, filled with humour, self-awareness and intelligence. Whose perspective is the one we should be paying more attention to? The one who experiences life as a disabled person? Or the one who views disability through a lens of deficits, loss and suffering, who compares an autistic person to a neurotypical person and finds them wanting?

Medical model vs social model of disability

It's important to understand how feelings about being a carer are shaped by the way society views disabled and chronically ill people. It can give us insight into some of the difficult feelings we may experience as someone we love becomes or is born disabled.

The medical model, which has prevailed as the dominant way of viewing disability, links disability to an individual's body. It assumes that a disability reduces a person's quality of life and the aim is to diminish, correct or cure that disability. The main focus is therefore on medical professionals to fix and improve functions so that a disabled person can lead as 'normal' a life as possible. The disabled person must strive as much as possible to conform to normative values. This is the model most of us who are non-disabled have come to know disability through. It is the way almost all our cultural understanding of disability is framed. From a carer's perspective, we may be expected to 'fix' the people we support and we too must strive towards a life that looks as 'normal' as possible. But there is another way of looking at disability and chronic illness.

The social model of disability identifies exclusion, negative attitudes and systemic barriers as the main reasons why a disabled person might not be able to participate fully in society. The simplest example of this is a wheelchair user not being able to fully access a building through the use of ramps and lifts. The wheelchair is not the problem, the lack of ramps and lifts is. But it is not just about physical access. It puts the focus on society to address changes that need to be made to accommodate the lives of people who have all kinds of disabilities. This might include not underestimating a person's quality of life, providing sufficient social support, providing information in many formats (such as Braille and audio), providing physical access and even flexible working hours to take into account health problems that might occur alongside an impairment or disability.

The social model does not deny that certain impairments will come with a lot of physical challenges. Chronic pain, for instance, or anxiety, might make a condition hard to live with. The point of the social model, however, is not to layer more unnecessary difficulties onto a person who has an impairment or disability, but to make sure that the environment and society does not prevent them from living the full life they wish to have. From the point of view of a carer, the social model allows us to look to what is controllable, for instance accessing public transport or getting social care support, rather than focusing on what is uncontrollable: the impairment itself.

The problem with the word 'carer'

When I contacted Natalie Lee about her experiences raising her 10-year-old daughter who has a visual impairment, she confessed that she was surprised. She struggled to view herself as a carer, even though, logically, she could see that she was one. Her daughter's visual impairment had meant adaptations to family life. Her emotional needs, as a child with a degenerative eye condition who will one day lose her sight completely, have been significant. But the word carer, she explained, evoked a deep discomfort. She associated it with victim and rescuer, which she said didn't feel good at all.

Natalie was not the only person I spoke to who revealed the uncomfortable feelings that the word carer brought up in them. Dr Frances Ryan, a British journalist who has written extensively about disability rights and culture, told me that while we should be able to see a word such as carer in a neutral way, the fact remains that in our society, with disabled and chronically ill people so devalued, to be a carer is a loaded term. Natalie associating the term carer with rescuer is not an unusual. It comes from a cultural idea that disabled people are victims, have no autonomy and must be looked after by non-disabled people.

Ruth Ridgeway, whose partner Steve has a spinal injury from a fall five years ago, also expressed discomfort at the term. Ruth felt the term 'carer' took away from Steve's autonomy and would lead others to believe he was completely dependent on her. She saw carers as people who tend to another's entire personal care needs, such as feeding and bathing. Steve uses a wheelchair and is far from physically dependent on Ruth. He manages all his own personal care needs and gets around independently. The couple prefer to use the word 'support' when it comes to the way they manage things between them in the household. The support Ruth provides varies according to what's going on with Steve's health at the time. His spinal injury has left him with chronic nerve pain which can severely affect his ability to sleep at times. Other aspects of his injury, such as needing to use a catheter, are time-consuming. Ruth takes on a larger share of the household responsibilities such as cooking, cleaning and food shopping so that Steve can manage his energy. She also takes on much of the financial responsibilities. Steve runs his own business but there have been times when his health has had to come first, and the business has taken a back seat, leaving Ruth to provide the majority of their income. This is not easy and, at times, has put a lot of pressure on Ruth. But as far as both Ruth and Steve are concerned, that's not caring, that's supporting your partner.

Dr Ryan said that in her years interviewing disabled people, support is by far a preferred term to care. She herself only uses the word carer in relation to parents looking after disabled children. The association with complete dependence that comes with the word carer she feels is appropriate in regards to children. Which probably explains why I don't feel uncomfortable using the term in relation to my son. Whether it's right or wrong for us to have so many negative and narrow views of the word, language is vitally important, especially amongst a community that has been so marginalised. Caring for someone is providing them with support. But perhaps it will take a dismantling of the negative views of disability on a much wider scale before we can use the terms 'care' and 'carer' freely without negative connotations.

In 2018 Sara Gibbs, a TV comedy writer, took to Twitter to set a few things straight about her experiences of being cared for. Sara was finally given an autism diagnosis at the age of 30 after years of struggling with many things others seemed to find straightforward. She wrote how she is often dismissed by parents of autistic kids as not being able to understand the struggles their children go through because she has a prominent and successful career and is highly verbal. In a long thread, Sara detailed all that her husband did to support her that allowed her to continue working. When I spoke to her, she confirmed that he did pretty much every single thing for their household, including all the shopping, cooking and cleaning, as well as being in complete charge of their social lives. It gave Sara the cognitive space to work and, without his support, she says that there is no way she would be able to write at the level she does. She believes that it is right and fair to talk openly about what a difference having support can make for a disabled person. For her it's the difference between a thriving career and not being able to work at all. Her husband is also her carer and she feels that's nothing to be ashamed of.

While the term 'carer' implies unidirectional support in our current culture, caring for someone isn't necessarily a one-way street, even when it involves a high level of personal care. My son might need me to keep him physically safe and structure his environment to make it more manageable for him, but he provides me with endless affection, laughter and a completely unique perspective on the world. Ruth Ridgeway might necessarily handle the household chores and take over their life and business admin when Steve is experiencing high levels of pain but Steve, to give a couple of examples, provides Ruth with incredible emotional support, does all the driving and is excellent company. This might be the case in many couples regardless of disability. Sara Gibbs relies on her husband John to do much of the detailed work of their lives, but John regularly reminds Sara that she's much better than he is at big-picture thinking. Support is not a one-way street.

Another way of looking at disability

What happens when we look at disability, not through the narrative of tragedy, loss and pity but one of ordinary nuanced life, with both ups and downs?

Kieran and Michelle Rose sat around their kitchen table with me drinking tea while they explained the story of their youngest daughter Livvy's autism diagnosis. Far from the fearful, sadness-filled reference to D-Day (as many parents online refer to the day of their child's diagnosis), the Rose family, at Livvy's request, turned it in to a celebration. Kieran, an autism consultant and writer, was diagnosed as autistic when he was 23 years old, and the eldest of their three children, Quinn, was diagnosed aged seven. The family had known for a long time that Livvy was also autistic, but as she was hyperlexic (the ability to read and use language far above your age), having taught herself to read by playing Minecraft when she was two, and highly academically able (she has a genius level IQ), doctors and teachers were reluctant to assess her despite her extremely high levels of anxiety. In fact, the biggest worry they had when they went for the follow-up appointment was that she would be refused a diagnosis. Livvy excitedly requested a cake and a party to celebrate the news that she would soon be able to identify as autistic just like her dad and eldest brother. That afternoon, after they left the doctor's office with Livvy's official diagnosis, she said to her dad: 'So I'm autistic now like you?' and Kieran replied, 'You've always been autistic, it's just now other people know that you are.' They went home to celebrate with cake. At six years old, Livvy saw autism as a positive thing and diagnosis was a validation of the many challenges she faced that her neurotypical peers did not.

This is far from the typical story of an autism diagnosis. There aren't many families that have openly embraced their neurodivergence so completely that the diagnosis itself is cause for celebration. And there is a reason that most families can't do this right now and that's down to the medical model of disability framing autism around deficits rather than difference, which is how the Roses view it. Kieran would be the first to tell you that this doesn't mean being autistic doesn't come with huge challenges. He has spent his adult life in a cycle of recurrent burnout, caused largely by masking his autistic tendencies and trying to go about life as if he is neurotypical. He is well aware of the challenges that his children will face. But the family see autism as an integral part of who they are. Autism is neither a 'good' or a 'bad' thing. It just is. The Rose children who are autistic have both extra challenges and extra skills. The challenges can be quite intense and require adaptation and support that aren't always easy. But that doesn't mean that either Kieran or Michelle (who is not autistic) wish their children were neurotypical. The children are the way they are and they couldn't imagine trying to change them or fight against that. What they see is their responsibility as parents is providing support appropriate to each child, no matter what that child's needs are.

Role models

There is no doubt in my mind that having a parent with the same disability is going to be an advantage to any disabled child. Seeing a parent manage their impairments or disability, advocate for themselves and go about their lives using adaptations, means those things will always be normal. But for many disabled children, or newly disabled adults, these role models are missing and need to be sought out. Could the better representation of disabled people in mainstream media go some way to help this?

When her daughter Natty was around a year old, Hayley Newman was stopped in her tracks while shopping in her local Cornish town. In the large window display of a surf shop was a photo of a young child with Down's syndrome, modelling some children's clothing. It turned out that it was the child of the brand owners. It was the first time Hayley had really realised she had never seen any child with Down's syndrome, let alone any other disabled child, modelling before. She decided it was time for that to change and she went about contacting as many local brands as possible to ask if they would consider using her daughter for a campaign. Frugi, an organic children's clothing brand, took Hayley up on the offer and Natty modelled in their next campaign. It made national headlines and Hayley and Natty were invited onto live morning TV to talk about it. Natty went on to be the first child with Down's syndrome to be featured in a national 'Back to School' campaign.

The same day that Hayley and I spoke on the phone I had popped into a prominent high-street brand to buy a few pairs of leggings for my daughter. As I walked past the boy's department I glanced around and smiled. The in-store posters featured an array of kids of all races as well as a boy with skin pigmentation differences. Hayley and I couldn't help but laugh about how far the fashion industry has come since her now 13-year-old daughter made it onto national TV for appearing in one ad. Things are changing slowly, but there is a long way to go.

Emma Gardner is a creative director at a leading London creative agency, and mother to five-year-old Dotty, who has a rare genetic condition. After feeling angry and sad at the time of her diagnosis, Emma realised that her difficult feelings about it were largely a societal problem. She started asking more difficult questions at work. Why aren't we talking about disability? Why do people tilt their heads in pity when they see my daughter in a wheelchair? Where are the positive stories around disability and why are disabled people so hidden? She feels extremely fortunate that her daughter has given her the opportunity to ask some really challenging questions of her industry. Emma has since organised industry events around disability, representation and inclusion in media. It's scary, she admits, because we don't want to get the language wrong, or make mistakes, especially as someone who doesn't have lived experience as a disabled person. But that becomes part of the problem, if nobody is willing to stand up and say 'why aren't we talking about this?' Emma says for her this realisation came through having a disabled child, but when she runs an event, she sees the same revelations on people's faces when it dawns on them that they haven't even considered asking the questions about disability and representation. She says: 'We are all walking around, these supposedly really educated people, and we are not even considering it.' Emma still has one relative who tears up every time she sees Dotty, and mutters about how sad it is. Emma has had to be firm with her and tell her that it must stop. But she also knows media are to blame for the opinions that affect her daughter's life daily, and she is determined to be part of the solution.

Traditionally in mainstream media, disabled people have not been viewed as whole humans, worthy of being seen for their common humanity, but instead singled out because of their perceived deficits. Most of us can remember watching hours-long telethons, with story after story of children overcoming insurmountable difficulties to inspire the non-disabled folk at home to part with their hard-earned cash for charity. The author Shane Burcaw describes his own experience of being wheeled out in front of the cameras aged eight for this exact purpose. Burcaw, who has spinal muscular atrophy, agreed to appear on the Muscular Dystrophy Association (MDA) Labor Day Telethon which brought in millions of dollars to fund research every year. In front of a live audience and with millions of people at home watching, he felt the shame of being described as dreaming of running on the playground with friends and being free of the wheelchair that held him back. Shane couldn't recognise the person the host was describing. He had never spent any time wanting to walk. His chair took him everywhere he needed to go. The host had made it sound like he spent all day in his bedroom crying. It was the first time Shane had seen how the world saw him. Someone to be pitied. Someone living a hopeless and depressing life. And it was done to raise money. He goes on to describe how old ladies would approach his mother in the super-market to give their condolences. Shane, who is an incredibly funny writer, thinks this is the root of his sense of humour, developed as he grew his thick skin. He writes: 'Society had it wrong, but the wrongness was so deeply ingrained from centuries of outcasting the disabled that it didn't help to get angry. Once again it was easier to laugh.'[34] Disability does not equal sadness, he goes on to say. But if our entire view of disability is through a non-disabled lens, this is the story we are sold.

Inspiration porn

It was Australian activist and comedian Stella Young who coined the term 'inspiration porn'. In a 2014 Ted Talk, Stella, who is a wheelchair user, tells the story of doing her teacher training rounds and being interrupted by a Year-11 boy halfway through the class to ask her when she was going to start her inspirational speech. She explains that this boy, just like most non-disabled people, had only encountered disability as an inspiration. She says: 'We have been lied to. We have been sold the idea that disability is a Bad Thing. Capital B capital T. And to live with disability makes you exceptional. It's not a bad thing. And it doesn't make you exceptional.'[35]

Inspiration porn is the objectification of disabled people for the benefit of non-disabled people. It's in memes and videos that get shared online, showing a disabled person getting on with their lives but for the purpose of non-disabled people to feel better about themselves. Videos like those showing a baby having her hearing aids put on for the first time, or a paraplegic groom being held up by friends on his wedding day so that he can dance with his bride. The purpose of these widely shared videos is to make non-disabled people feel inspired, while the disabled person becomes the object through which the story is told. This could also be through a non-disabled character acting as rescuer to a passive disabled character, like the stories of the popular, non-disabled kid in high school being treated as a hero for asking a disabled kid to the prom. Or like at the 2020 Oscars, when Shia Labeouf was praised as a 'great guy' in the media for sharing a stage with his *Peanut Butter Falcon* co-star Zack Gottsagen, simply because Zack has Down's syndrome.

How many times have you viewed images of a disabled person and been told, either indirectly or directly, that 'your excuse is not valid', the implication being that if a disabled person is capable of something, then you as a non-disabled person have no excuse not to also be capable of doing it? Non-disabled people are invited to compare themselves to disabled people and to come out thinking that however bad things are, at least they are not them. Inspiration porn is so embedded in our cultural understanding of disability that it bleeds over into the lives of those who support disabled people.

Morris writes that disabled people face undermining messages each day about their value in the world. I would argue that part of the reason that carers struggle with the weight of some of their responsibilities is the same. We live in a society obsessed with productivity and output. If we don't value the lives of disabled people, we can't expect to be valued as someone who supports a disabled person. If we are surrounded by messages that tell us disabled people are only there to make us feel better about our own lives, what happens when our partner or parent becomes disabled and we become their carer? The messages we have received our whole lives, that disability is one of the worst things that could happen to us, takes over and we are layered with unnecessary sorrow.

Intersections

The direct and indirect discrimination against disabled people can be compounded when you add further intersections. 30% of families with a disabled family member are living in poverty.[36] Whether that's lack of appropriate access and support within the work place, or lack of paid carers, or the lack of flexibility that both a disabled person or a carer may need from an employer, then working – or working as many hours as you would like – becomes challenging. The costs of being disabled or raising a disabled child are also high, with an average of £550 a month being spent on costs related to a disability. Poverty brings further problems to families who might already to struggling to access opportunities and be out and about in the community.

If you are not a home owner, for instance, other problems arise. One mother I spoke to who has two autistic children, one of whom has severe learning difficulties, was recently evicted from her private rental. Their flat was on the first floor and when her son had trouble sleeping in the night he would jump up and down repeatedly. Eventually, the landlord evicted them after the downstairs neighbour kept complaining. They were put into inappropriate emergency accommodation for months, which was extremely distressing for the children. When the council finally came back with a property that would be more permanent, they had completely ignored the reason for the eviction and had given them a first-floor flat. As this mother cried in the housing office, explaining her son's behaviour and needs, she was told that only wheelchair users were given ground-floor flats, and her son was not a wheelchair user. Eventually, after many more months and arguments, the family were given a more appropriate short-term home. Many families with a disabled family member, despite what is commonly believed, may wait years and years for housing that is accessible and meets their needs. Years where many rooms in a house are inaccessible to the disabled person and where a carer must carry them to access a bathroom or bedroom where a wheelchair and other equipment cannot go. There are currently 1.8 million disabled people with unmet housing needs in the UK.[37]

Though it may be easy to imagine how strained finances add to the difficulty of caring, racism can also add pressures. Stacey Leigh, whose son is autistic, told me that as a black mother raising a black son, she worries constantly about what will happen if her son behaves inappropriately in front of police. Since he was two years old she has been trying to teach him about the importance of always stopping and listening to police if they speak to him, using toy police cars to try and get the message across. Being black and not responding in an expected way may be far more risky than being white in the same situation.

Marva is the mother of an 11-year-old boy, Liondo, who attends the same school as Arthur. We often swap information about disability allowance forms, benefits and ideas for Christmas gifts and days out for our boys, who have lots of similarities and shared interests. Marva, who is originally from Jamaica, has experienced quite different responses from strangers in public than Arthur and I have. Liondo is tall for his age and has dark black skin. During a meltdown they sometimes get outright hostility. Waiting for a bus one day someone even hit Liondo, claiming that he was behaving aggressively towards them. Marva is certainly facing more challenges raising a black disabled child than I am in raising a light-skinned one. The barriers that exist for people of colour are compounded by the ableism that is also rife in our society.

When I began to see that I might have been misguided in my ideas about what my son's life would be like as a disabled person, I could filter out the real fears from the imagined. And I do have very real fears. I worry about government funding that is stripping specialist education to the bone. I worry about a social care system that is inadequate and is leaving far too much in the hands of unpaid carers, with very real consequences. The 2018 Learning Disability Mortality Review Programme (LeDeR) conducted by Bristol University spells out one of my greatest fears. That based on the average, my son is likely to die 20 years before his non-disabled peers from a preventable cause, simply because he has a learning disability.[38] These are not imagined fears and they terrify me. But the same problem is at the root of them. That society refuses to see disabled people as of equal value to non-disabled people. Addressing my own ingrained ableism is the beginning of fighting for my son's right to equitable access to education, to opportunities, to quality healthcare and to social care support. I cannot do this without admitting to myself that I was once a person who both feared and pitied those with learning disabilities.

Shane Burcaw writes: 'From the earliest days I can remember, my body, society, and the world around me have been feeding me the same message: You are sick and different and your existence is a pity. People are programmed to feel bad for me, knowing nothing about the quality of my life. At times, the outside perception that my life is negative and sad became so powerful that I internalised it and developed harmful beliefs that I was a burden to even the people who love me most.'[39]

As carers we have an extremely important role to play in challenging these negative perceptions. It is not about denying the difficulties of living with an impairment or chronic illness, or pretending life is a bed of roses. It's about recognising that the lives of disabled people are just as valid, just as varied and just as full as those of non-disabled people.

As an inherently optimistic person, I can imagine a different society. One in which a new mother is congratulated by the midwife when her baby with Down's syndrome is born. When someone who has spinal injury doesn't have to worry about how they'll get to and from work because the public transport is accessible and their office is too. Where a person with a visual impairment has plenty of employers willing to make adaptations so they can join the team. Imagine if a newly disabled person could just concentrate on adapting to their impairment rather than face prejudice and exclusion from society.

In such a world, being a carer would be a far less scary prospect. One in which the role was not pitied or put on a pedestal but accepted as a natural part of life. It wouldn't fix our frequent sleepless nights or make chronic pain less difficult to witness. But how much energy could be saved if we didn't have to argue and fight for our loved ones' most basic rights? And how much sorrow could be avoided if we challenged the notion that to be disabled is among the worst things that could happen to you?

CHAPTER 4

Expectations

'*This is not how your story ends. It's simply where it takes a turn you didn't expect.*'[40]

Cheryl Strayed, memoirist, novelist and essayist

When Mary Susan and Sean McConnell filled out their adoption paperwork they decided not to tick the box that said they were interested in a child with additional needs. At 26 years old they thought they barely knew anything about having children as it was, let alone a disabled child. But by chance the agency they were using sent them through a child via email who did not meet their criteria. It gave the details of a one-year-old girl living in an orphanage in Ghana. Something about this child caught both their attentions and they immediately knew she was meant to be part of their family. The agency were clear: she had a diagnosis of cerebral palsy but there would be no more details than that. Were they up for such an unknown future? Mary Susan and Sean surprised themselves by their answer. They were absolutely up for it and planned their first visit to meet the baby girl that they would go on to name Abiella.

When Mary Susan and I first discussed what the adoption process was like, I had assumed they knew the full extent of Abiella's disabilities. She said that, actually, it was almost the opposite. Before their first trip to Ghana, they made a visit to the paediatrician at their local hospital to ask about the kind of information they should be trying to obtain. The doctor told them that with so little information on her it was best to assume every kind of profound disability, until they knew for sure. She taught them some tips for getting an idea if she was visually impaired, deaf or had any muscle and limb control. On that first visit they spent each afternoon in the shade of a large tree in the orphanage gardens, getting to know Abiella. One afternoon a car parked nearby and the door slammed loudly. Abiella jumped and Sean and Mary Susan cheered as they knew for sure that she had some hearing. Rather than looking at each impairment as a loss, each clue as to her ability to respond to them and the environment around her felt like gathering knowledge about her. They didn't yet know whether Abiella could see but they could use their voices to communicate with her till they knew more. It was on their third visit, almost a year later, that they were able to bring Abiella home to Tennessee, still unsure of the full extent of her disabilities.

It is the way that they both looked at Abiella's needs as simply how things were for her rather than as losses which is most striking about Mary Susan and Sean. We live in a culture that insists on viewing disability in terms of loss. But they chose to take the opposite view, as well as choosing a more challenging path into parenthood. When women are pregnant it's not uncommon to hear the phrase, 'we don't care what the gender is, as long as it's healthy.' But what if our children aren't born healthy or non-disabled? What if our partners, siblings or parents become disabled or acquire chronic illnesses? Can we really always expect for life to deliver us a smooth road? Bodies and minds that remain free from impairment?

Rita Eichenstein, a Los Angeles-based paediatric neuropsychologist who specialises in working with families with what she describes as atypical children, explains that in her experience it is our expectations that cause our suffering after an unexpected diagnosis. In her book *Not What I Expected*, she says that understanding our personal and cultural expectations – really examining them – is an important step towards being able to let them go. A story from one of her clients, Ora, who was the mother of a young child with a terminal condition, as well as a hospice care worker, illustrates her point well. Ora tells her: 'Imagine if infants were born ready to use the potty and diapering wasn't the norm of our expectations. If you gave birth to a baby who needed diapers, it would be considered a tragedy. The fact that you would have to change diapers for the first two years of life would be seen as a devastating concept. But every parent is able to change their baby's diapers. Why? Because it is the natural state of affairs.'[41]

When there is a mismatch between our expectations and our reality, we suffer. It is natural and human to feel sad, angry, confused, fearful and resentful when this happens. We all have expectations, whether we are conscious of them or not. We may be about to enjoy the peace and freedom of being an empty nester, when an elderly parent becomes too unwell to manage alone. Or perhaps about to take a job abroad when our partner develops a chronic illness that makes this impossible. Becoming a carer also means changes within a relationship. A married couple where one suddenly becomes much more dependent on the other. An elderly parent who must leave their own home and move in with one of their children, after a lifetime of being the head of their own household. Though we may accept that these could be possibilities in our future, they still may not sit easily alongside our expectations for our lives. They require huge adjustments on everyone's part. But it is possible to adjust and eventually let go of our expectations over time. To discover a new normal.

Ora explained to Rita that her acceptance of her daughter's condition was down to her ability to not only let go of expectations but also of her ego. Rita writes that the two are often connected. Our egos can cause us difficulty by expecting our situation to be different to how it is, and by expecting that we can control our situation. If we are, for instance, caught out by our parent's bladder suddenly losing control in public, we can either view it as an unfortunate situation that is part of the condition they have, or we might be overwhelmed with embarrassment. Our embarrassment can lead to resentment and anger, as our brains rage at the injustice of such a thing happening. It's not that it's wrong or unnatural to feel those things, but we end up suffering more than we need to. It is by no means easy, but it is possible to reframe our expectations.

Feelings of loss

Unlike Mary Susan and Sean McConnell, I *did* see my son's diagnosis as a loss at first. In the months after his official diagnosis, while hurriedly trying to piece together ways to support him, I also spent time dwelling on the things that may never be. He might never speak, tell me what he dreamt at night, what he did in school that day or even if he was in pain. I had no idea that I'd even had the expectation that I would have a child who could tell me where something hurt, until I had a child who couldn't. Many of our expectations are unconscious and unknown to us, until they are unmet. We take for granted that a child will walk and talk, but this isn't a given. Not long before his diagnosis Arthur said his first couple of words. I told a friend who had older kids that he'd started speaking. She laughed at the relief in my voice and said, 'of course he's started speaking, did you think he would get to 18 and not speak?' In her world, she could take development for granted and assumed everyone else could too.

Rita Eichenstein explains that while other animals experience grief for actual loss, as humans we are the only species to experience grief for abstract loss. The loss of things that never were. The loss of expectations – whether that's expecting your child would speak or that your partner would be able to travel the world with you after the kids left home but is now too ill to do so. This is due to our unique ability to dwell on what might have been and worry about what is still to come.

In the early days of Arthur's diagnosis I felt an avalanche of extreme emotions. As I tried to pick them apart, distinguish them and understand them, it became clearer. I did feel a sense of loss. I was terrified, for all the same reasons Jess Wilson explained she found herself retching over a toilet bowl (see Chapter 3, page 74) that my son was part of a minority group that was marginalised, ignored and often abused. I was also sad about saying goodbye to the imaginary life that I had not even realised I had constructed in my mind. The life where I would take my children on a plane to visit our family in Australia. The life where Arthur would tell me jokes and tease his little sister mercilessly, just as my brothers had done to me. The life where my son would speak fluently, meet expected academic targets for his age and have a huge array of choices in his future. These are things that had never been and, although I remain very open-minded about what his future holds, may never be. It was an abstract loss but the feelings were very real.

It would be easy to dismiss these feeling of abstract loss as small and insignificant compared to actual loss. But the loss of a future you imagined can be as overwhelmingly significant as the loss of something very real and tangible. At first, knowing all the challenges my son would face in his life felt as large and heavy in my heart as my mother's death. I was not sad because he was different. I was broken by the idea that he would have to struggle all his life to do things that most of us take for granted. And I was terrified I wouldn't be able to do a good enough job of supporting him.

But as Rita Eichenstein explains: 'What exactly has been lost? The fantasy of the perfect child.' As I began to understand that, the process of beginning to let go of that fantasy became possible. I realised I had no interest in an imaginary child. I wanted my living, breathing, giggling, shouting, whirlwind of a child who was right there in front of me.

The use of the word grief in relation to a family member becoming or being born disabled is commonplace. In his article 'Do Not Mourn For Us', autistic writer and advocate Jim Sinclair appeals to parents to 'grieve if you must, for your own lost dreams. But do not mourn *us*. We are alive. We are real. And we are waiting here for you.'[42] The Merriam-Webster dictionary definition of grief is 'a deep and poignant distress caused by or as if by bereavement'.[43] With its inextricable link with death and mourning, it is understandable that many disabled adults get angry at the word when used to describe feelings about a disabled family member. This is a complicated and messy topic. As Jim Sinclair acknowledges, there is a loss in expectations which must be addressed and moved through. For some the word grief describes perfectly the overwhelming sadness that a loved one, whether a child or a partner or parent, will experience physical pain or emotional distress, or struggle with daily tasks because of their impairment or disability. For others it might be that the sense of loss accompanies the realisation that there are things in life outside of their control.

I think that Jim Sinclair expresses it well when he asks parents not to 'mourn for us'. Grief refers to the inward experience and feelings around loss, while mourning is an outward expression of those feelings. Over the years I have read the words of many disabled adults who say how difficult it was to witness their parents mourning for the child they expected to have. How hard it was to accept themselves and their disabled bodies when their parents could not. Safe exploration of these intense feelings when someone we love receives a life-changing diagnosis is essential if we are to adjust our expectations. We need to understand what these feelings are and where they come from in order to move through them. In my own case it was about understanding my fears for my son's future and for his emotional and physical wellbeing. My fears, for instance, that a serious illness would be missed because he couldn't communicate well or that he would be hit by a car during a sudden panic near a busy road. Of course, many carers are in a situation where the child, parent or partner they are supporting has a life-limiting condition and I explore that aspect of loss and grief in the next chapter.

Every person will have different reasons and beliefs, both cultural and personal, which will make up the myriad of feelings that accompany such a life-changing experience. If we can unpick these, either alone, with a therapist, close friend or support group, these feelings won't hold so much sway over us. We can let them go.

Rita says that in all her years of experience working with families she can see that the emotional impact a parent carer has on their child is directly related to how well they understand and process their own feelings and reactions.[44] In other words, what is good for a carer's mental wellbeing is also good for their child, their partner or parent.

Perspective

Syreeta and Rob were both living and working in Hong Kong when they met and fell in love. Rob was in advertising, working for large international brands, and Syreeta was a product designer. They were living a fast-paced life doing work they loved. While on a holiday in Sydney, Syreeta woke early one morning to find Rob stumbling around the hotel room, in pain and unable to respond to her. She called an ambulance, and when they arrived at the hospital it became clear that Rob was fighting for his life, after experiencing a major brain haemorrhage. After 12 hours of brain surgery, the neurosurgeon told Syreeta that Rob was alive but in a coma, and his injuries were likely to be devastating. All they could do was wait and see.

With no home to go to, Syreeta stayed by Rob's side, sleeping in the hospital and waiting for his mother and sister to arrive from the UK. After three weeks he came out of the coma, unable to speak, stand or hold a pen. It would take another three months before Rob was well enough to travel back to the UK. In one swift moment, they had both lost their home in Hong Kong, their jobs and their income. Rob had lost his ability to communicate and all of his independence, not knowing what he could gain back. Syreeta was now a full-time carer, living with Rob's parents, whom she had only met a handful of times, in a part of the UK she had never lived and where she knew no one. Syreeta told me that it was the collection of losses that had been so untethering. Not one single part of their life was recognisable from one moment to the next. They had to completely redesign their lives from scratch.

When I spoke to Syreeta and Rob on the phone from their new home in Somerset, their baby boy Grayson was gurgling and sneezing in Syreeta's lap. It is five years since Rob's brain injury and life looks very different to how it looked before. When Rob was seen by a neurologist back in the UK, they were astounded by what they saw. Rob should have died that day; his life had been saved by an incredibly determined team in Sydney. It had taken Syreeta three attempts to find a rehabilitation centre that would take Rob, in order to get him well enough to travel back to the UK. The first two said his injuries were so severe he wasn't worth rehabilitating. The third one was run by a young doctor and, shocked by Rob's age (he was in his thirties at the time), they admitted him and helped him gain enough strength in order for an airline to admit him on a plane.

Since then, they have gone from a Lincolnshire hospital, to Syreeta supporting Rob full time at his parents' home, to getting married, starting a business together, moving across the country and welcoming their baby boy into the world. Rob's recovery has been slow and hard work. He still struggles with his speech and movement. The nature of brain injuries mean that each day can be completely different. They have both had to slow their lives down to a snail's pace in comparison to the life they had been leading before Rob's injury. But what it most astounding about Syreeta and Rob's story is not only what they have achieved together in his recovery and their family life, but their firm belief that, despite all they lost, they both truly believe they have gained so much along the way.

There is a lot of science behind why people like Syreeta and Rob, despite their challenges and losses, lead lives that are happy and that they're incredibly proud of. It is the same science that explains why I find I have adjusted to life raising a disabled child.

As humans, it turns out we are pretty terrible at predicting what will make us happy. We have a lot of natural biases that mean we end up 'mis-wanting', as Daniel Gilbert, Harvard Professor of Psychology, puts it.[45] Certain things we think will make us very happy, and for the long term, don't actually make us that much happier and for hardly any time at all. On the flip side, when we try to predict how a negative experience will affect us, we think we will be utterly miserable and for a really long period of time, when in fact it will only make us a bit unhappy and not for so long. It's called impact bias and we are all prone to it.

Most of us have heard that more money, beyond a certain income, won't make us much happier. Part of the reason for this is hedonic adaptation. This is the fact that as humans, we are very adaptable and constantly adjust to our current circumstances. So while more money or a new car or house might feel great for a short while, we naturally adapt to our new circumstances and go back to how we were feeling before. The really interesting thing is that impact bias has an even stronger effect on how we think about negative events, where we think something bad happening to us will make us more miserable and for longer than it does. Humans are not just good at adjusting to so called 'good' things, we are also extremely good at adjusting to difficult things. According to Daniel Gilbert, we tend to be unaware of our ability to be resilient. And humans are extremely resilient.

According to research by Sonja Lyubomirsky of the University of California, circumstances only make up about 10% of what influences our happiness. That means income level, marriage and divorce, bereavement, health and disability actually have a fairly minimal effect on our happiness. Around 50% is set by our genes, which leaves around 40% of our happiness down to our actions and thoughts.[46] Though these numbers are disputed by some, there are many studies that show we have some influence over our happiness. We can have control over our thoughts and actions in a way we can't over much of our circumstances. It takes effort, but we can change the way we think and act to make us happier – even in challenging circumstances.

Mary Susan and Sean's daughter Abiella has profound disabilities that many parents in similar situations spend years grieving over. Although they hadn't planned to adopt a disabled child, as soon as they knew about Abiella, they quickly adjusted their expectations of parenthood to include her impairments. This included the expectation that they wouldn't know exactly what her future would look like. When they first brought her home, they were pleased to discover that she had no signs of seizures, which are common with Abiella's particular impairments. This unfortunately didn't last and she had her first seizure aged three, which was traumatic for them all.

They have had to deal with their share of terrifying ambulance rides, surgeries and new challenges, just as many parents of disabled children must. What they haven't dealt with is feeling that they have missed out on a non-disabled child. The ability to adjust their expectations has meant there is no additional suffering on top of the usual fears and worries about caring for their disabled child. The same is true for carers who adjust to their partner's or parent's sudden and unexpected impairments.

Another way in which our expectations can trip us up and cause us pain is we are not very good at evaluating things objectively. Our brains use reference points to judge how we *should* feel about things. This has been well illustrated in studies like the silver medal effect.[47] Psychologists studied gold, silver and bronze medal winners' facial expressions at multiple Olympic games and the results were not what most people expect. While the gold medallists were very happy with their result, the silver medallists were mostly very unhappy. The silver medallists came so close to winning gold, their reference point became that they missed out. On the other hand, bronze medallists narrowly missed receiving no medal at all, so were extremely pleased with their result. Despite the fact bronze is objectively not as good a result as silver, they were happier. The difference is the reference point each medallist measures themselves against. You could liken the McConnells to bronze medallists, and parents who are stuck on the fact they 'missed out' on a non-disabled child as silver medallists, who may be missing the fact they are still holding a medal.

We use reference points constantly to know how to judge a situation, and we do it mostly unconsciously. Our minds aren't particularly good at picking reference points either. An excellent example of this is a social comparison experiment where people are offered the choice of earning $100,000 while their co-workers earn $250,000, or choosing a salary of $50,000 and their co-workers will earn $25,000. In around half the cases people choose to earn $50,000 less if it means they earn double what everyone else is earning.[48]

But we can deliberately change our reference points. This is one of the really effective ways we can adjust how we choose to view our circumstances. When Syreeta was telling me the story of Rob's injury, it became really clear to me that their reference point for what a good life is has changed. Although they have had to deal with intense feelings of loss and sadness over what they both describe as a traumatic experience, they aren't comparing life today with life in Hong Kong, before the injury. They're comparing it to the other possibility. That Rob should have died that day. Although it hasn't been easy adjusting to life as a new mother whilst also supporting Rob, Syreeta said she doesn't feel the frustration and difficulties in the same way that she sees other new mothers express on social media. 'I just feel so lucky that I even get to do the laundry for my family,' she told me. A family that might not have existed.

Similarly, when I asked Rob what the challenges of accepting support from Syreeta had been, he struggled to answer the question. He told me it had been really challenging adjusting to his injuries, but when it came to Syreeta and all she had done to support him, he just felt lucky. The conversation the three of us had over Skype wasn't easy for Rob, so I sent some questions over to him via email and he and Syreeta recorded a voice message for me later, after Rob had had time to process the questions more. He teared up as he told Syreeta in the message: 'You've done everything and I imagine if it was just me . . . on my own . . . I'd have just gone.'

Syreeta has found a great sense of release in sharing their story, along with Rob, through writing, social media and a Ted Talk. Apart from being a wonderful way of connecting with others in similar situations, the sharing of the story itself acts as a reminder to them both of what could have been. They both have a deep sense of gratitude that they have come so far from that traumatic day and the even bigger loss that could have happened but didn't. This effect is called negative visualisation. One study has shown that couples who spent 15 minutes writing about if they had never met were much happier than couples who were simply asked to write about how they met.[49] By consciously reminding ourselves that we could lose what we have, we are able to better appreciate them. And when we appreciate what we have, it can negate much of the impact that negative life circumstances can bring. Gratitude is a widely recognised cognitive practice that has an extremely positive effect on our wellbeing.

Gratitude

What is gratitude exactly, and why does it work so well? In his book *Resilient*, Rick Hanson says that being grateful is not about denying feelings of loss and sadness, it's about looking at what is *also* true. You can experience difficulties *and* be grateful for what you have.[50] It's about appreciating what already is, not what was or what could be. Studies show that practising gratitude can have a beneficial effect on both our physical and mental health, with those who write down five things they are grateful for every day exercising more and feeling better about their lives.[51] Gratitude also works as an excellent antidote to social comparison. When we are consciously aware of the good things we have and the good people around us, whether that's because we write it down, talk about it, think about it or meditate on it, we don't tend to feel as envious of others.

It's important to note that, as authors Emily and Amelia Nagoski point out in their book *Burnout* that being told to 'be grateful' is often used as a weapon against women and marginalised groups to silence those who are expressing their suffering.[52] Being told to 'be grateful' that your disabled child even has a school place, when you are questioning whether their needs are being met, or that you should 'be grateful' that you get any social care support at all, when what you have is woefully inadequate, is not the kind of gratitude I'm talking about. It's no one else's place to tell you what you should be grateful for.

My conversation with Mary Susan was peppered with gratitude. Whether she has cultivated it consciously or has come to it naturally, either way Mary Susan tends to frame everything with a reference to gratitude. When she speaks about Abiella's seizures, she adds how lucky they are that they have been largely controllable. When Abiella experienced a period of extreme sensory processing difficulties that meant she became distressed going into new environments, they eventually discovered that it was probably triggered by an improvement in her eyesight. Yet another reason to be grateful. She speaks so highly and gratefully of all the medical staff who have supported their family over the years. When she reveals the story of one professional who was rude and acted as if Abiella wasn't in the room and spoke of her in terms of deficits, she reframed the experience as an excellent way of learning how to advocate for her daughter. She doesn't deny the difficult feelings when they go through a new challenge. She is scared and grateful, sad and grateful, angry and grateful. This is something we can all learn to cultivate.

One of the simplest and most effective ways to intentionally increase our gratitude is by keeping a notebook by the bed and each evening writing down a very short list of things you are grateful for in that moment. Rather than thinking about material things themselves, which can be ineffective for some, you can focus on who you are grateful for, and positive events.

You don't have to write things down, you can just bring your awareness to what you're grateful for. Every morning in the shower or on your commute to work, any time when you get a moment to yourself, you can bring your attention to the things that you appreciate. It sounds like too tiny a thing to make a difference but, as mentioned earlier, our brains are always underestimating what will make us feel better. Rick Hanson explains that by regularly bringing our attention to what we are grateful for, it hardwires it in our brains. You may need to begin with a habit of writing things down but, after some time, you may naturally be on the lookout for what you appreciate without much effort at all. It's also normal to need regular reminders to be conscious of what we are grateful for.

Comparison

Comparing ourselves to others is a natural function that developed in humans over millennia and served us well while living in small groups. But living in big communities and having access to far more people to compare ourselves with in both traditional and social media has meant this can have a very negative effect on us. On social media we are also comparing what someone is choosing to highlight to the world, with our own messy interior life. This is a terrible reference point. As we have already established, our brains are not very good at choosing reference points, but with conscious effort we can choose new ones.

Aside from the huge benefits of insight that I get from reading the work of disabled writers and following disabled people on social media, it has the other benefit of reminding me just how normal disability is. Online and in life, I know countless families that look like mine, where at least one of the children or one of the parents is disabled. Before I went to the conscious effort to seek them out, I was largely surrounded by non-disabled people, and my reference point was way off. Only a few years ago, most of my friends – including old school friends in Australia, work friends in London and new friends made through my children – were married, not disabled and raising non-disabled kids. I made the decision a while ago to make the effort to surround myself with all sorts of diverse friends and families and, as a result, my reference points are much more realistic.

We can go to a lot of effort to consciously change our reference points, but mainstream culture will often force comparisons upon us. Anyone who has a loved one who sees consultants in the NHS is well aware of the miserable way in which our letters are addressed to us. Underneath the name of the patient and their date of birth comes the heading PROBLEMS in bold letters followed by a list of diagnoses. Just there to remind us that we are not Normal but a Problem. It may sound like a tiny thing to someone who is outside of the world of disability, but the constant framing of an impairment or difference as a deficit to be fixed, cured or removed is a reminder that the medical model sees disability as a bad thing and non-disabled as normal.

Arthur spent his first three years of primary school in our local mainstream school. Although he was on an individualised curriculum, with learning outcomes developed in long meetings and implemented with the help of his own one-to-one support, for some unknown reason the school always sent me a standardised end-of-year report. He failed to meet every single of the criteria. All of them. It was like that classic joke of asking a fish to ride a bicycle. Each year I tore them up and threw them in the bin. At the end of his first year in a specialist ASD school, he received a detailed, personal and glowing report which compared him only to himself at the beginning of the school year. It was a wonderful reminder of why we chose for him to go to a specialist setting. A place where he is valued and treated as an individual, rather than included because he has to be. There is a huge amount of value in specialist schools, some of which is often ignored because mainstream is held up to be the best possible option. In my experience, the value that my son gets out of his school is far more than small class sizes and highly qualified and dedicated teachers. It is also in the attitude of normalcy with which disability is treated, with no child being compared to any other on standardised scales set by civil servants.

It takes effort to fight against these comparisons and expectations that are set from external mainstream culture. People will continue to impose their own views on us, to insist that our lives, or the lives of those we support, are of less value. When I had made the decision to actively pursue changing my son's school, an educational professional who works with disabled children asked me if I had 'resigned' myself to it. Another professional, after singing my daughter's praises, told me: 'You would never know she had a brother like Arthur at home.' I don't blame carers for feeling life is unfair in the face of this kind of prejudice. If we are going to get on with living our lives in the best way possible, we have to understand that these prejudices are not facts. They are ignorant opinions. The sooner we can distance ourselves from them and surround ourselves with those who share our values as well as sharing some of our life circumstances, the better things will be.

The psychology research scientist Sonja Lyubomirsky, as well as showing that gratitude for what we already have can make a huge difference to our wellbeing, also discovered that cultivating optimism had a similar effect. It is not, she writes, a way of denying difficulties and ignoring unfavourable information.[53] In fact, she says that optimists are very good at evaluating risks and are very aware of how positive outcomes are dependent on effort. If we are optimistic about our futures, we are more likely to be able to apply ourselves to the task of reaching our goals, and we are less likely to give up when we encounter hurdles.

I'm not sure if I have always been an optimist, or if it's something I cultivated over years of supporting my mother through difficult times. Either way, my experience with my mother showed me that extreme challenges can lead to incredibly positive things, as well as difficult things. That two things can be true at once. Things can be hard and beautiful, frightening and joyful. Perhaps this is why I had a feeling when Arthur was diagnosed that, despite how awful I felt in that moment, I knew somehow that eventually I would find a way to be ok with the challenges that were coming our way. It might sound horribly clichéd to say it, but I had already proven to myself I could do hard things. Somewhere inside me I knew I had the capacity to adjust my expectations of parenthood to include disability and possible life-long support. I'm extremely glad I felt optimistic that I could achieve that. In this way, I can be grateful for experiencing difficulties earlier on in my life with my mother, so that I had the perspective of life not always running smoothly when I became a parent to a disabled child.

Syreeta and Rob, though they are still dealing with the trauma of Rob's injury, are able to see the good things they have in their lives. This positive outlook is often referred to as post traumatic growth.[54] Post-traumatic growth is more likely to occur when we find meaning in the challenges that come our way. It can show up as a renewed belief in what we can endure, improved relationships, greater sense of compassion for others who suffer, and in developing a deeper more satisfying life philosophy.[55]

Syreeta and Rob were fairly early on in their relationship when Rob's brain injury happened. When they returned to the UK, Rob's mother took Syreeta aside and gave her an out. She told her she would understand if she needed to walk away. Although at the time Syreeta says she was angry and upset at the suggestion, she can now look back and see the compassion with which Rob's mother meant it. But Syreeta had no intentions of leaving. She loved Rob and to her there was no choice to make. They would spend their lives together, no matter if that life looked different to how they first imagined.

If I try to imagine what life would be like now, if Arthur hadn't been born disabled, I just can't see it. That imaginary boy, the one who speaks fluently and goes on sleepovers with friends and keeps me company on the flight to Australia, is long gone. He would be someone completely different, not my brilliant, funny Arthur. I cannot look at what we have been through together and wish it away. That's not to say at 4am after a hard night I don't have a cry and wish things were easier for him (and me). Sometimes I really do wish things were easier. Those moments pass, but the perspective of all that we have gained stays. Somehow, in the scheme of things, a bad night makes me savour the good ones. A delayed milestone makes it all the more precious. Knowing that we are doing ok when he can't hold a conversation certainly makes you far less concerned about piano lessons, exam results and competitive sports. Arthur is carving his own path and it is a relief not to have to think about him in relation to anyone else. There is a freedom in not doing what everyone else is doing.

Not long after Arthur's diagnosis, in the midst of my rush to research therapies that might support him, I came across a depressing read in an American newspaper. It was about a family who had gone $200,000 into debt to fund therapies for their now seven-year-old child, that weren't covered by their medical insurance. They had thrown a huge amount of money into private therapists, hoping that it would make all the difference. Their son was still non-speaking and they were in a financial crisis. They were devastated and told the journalist the best they could hope for was that their son would bag groceries at the supermarket. The article made me livid with rage. Firstly at the assumption that working at a supermarket was such a terrible thing, but also that the value they attached to their child was related to the job he would be able to manage as an adult. Not to mention a private therapy market feeding off the fears and worries of parents who are willing to bankrupt themselves to chase developmental milestones.

I have had people imply many times that they assume I have reduced my hopes and dreams for Arthur. That somehow, because of the challenges he faces, I don't have high expectations. But I have very high expectations for him. I want him to live a full, rich and adventurous life, with loving relationships and a sense of purpose that gets him out of bed each day. They are the same hopes and expectations that I have for my daughter. The way they will live their lives will, I'm sure, look very different. But I don't think either of their lives need to be any less fulfilling than the other. Any less filled with love than the other. They will simply be different.

CHAPTER 5

Grief

'*Our culture is imbued with the belief that we can fix just about anything and make it better; or, if we can't, that it's possible to trash what we have and start all over again. Grief is the antithesis of this belief; it eschews avoidance and requires endurance, and forces us to accept that there are some things in this world that simply cannot be fixed.*'[56]

Julia Samuel, psychotherapist and paediatric counsellor

It was around 9pm when I received the phone call. I had been in the shower and my hair was soaking wet. I had just enough time to throw on a dressing gown when I was told my dad was on the phone and needed to speak to me. Dad was working in Canada and I knew there had to be a really good reason why he was calling me during his working day. I heard the sob that escaped his mouth as he told me the news, and I began to shake and sob myself. This was it, I thought to myself. The moment I had been expecting for years. After I hung up, I wondered: is this how I was expecting to feel? Is this what I imagined it would be like? My dressing gown was soaked through and I couldn't stop shaking. I couldn't tell if it was the cold or the shock. Why now, I thought as I cried. Why not now, came the reply in my head.

Early the next morning I was standing on a freezing cold platform at Paddington Station, waiting for a train to the airport. It was a spot I strongly associated with a trip my family had made to London when I was seven. I'd been so excited to see the famous train station and the place where Paddington Bear was discovered and adopted by the Browns. It had always felt magical to me. Like the starting point of great adventure. Now as I waited, I saw a young family, a mother and two children who were about seven and eight years old. I watched as they chatted and laughed. I felt an immense sense of loss. My family as I knew it was gone. Now Paddington Station would remind me of that cold morning after my mother's death, flying home to her funeral. In that moment, clear as a bell in my mind, I knew I wanted to be a mother one day. I also knew that I wouldn't truly feel her loss until I was a mother myself.

I did a lot of grieving for my mum while she was still alive. Her death was by no means inevitable, as it is with some diseases, but her grip on life seemed precarious. It wasn't just that I was mentally preparing myself for her death. It was also a matter of the loss of my old mum. The mum who was present, who was reliable, who was a person I could turn to no matter what. She wasn't that mother any more and no amount of wishing would make it so. She was at times present and someone I could turn to. But I had lost the person I could count on and who could hold my feelings when life was difficult. I was her protector, rather than her daughter. That relationship was still precious to me and I was grateful for it, but it was not the mother/daughter relationship I had known in my early childhood.

On the one hand I knew that, after a few suicide attempts, her life was on a fine edge with the potential to tip over at any point. And on the other, that if she managed to hold on and stay with us she was never going to be the mother I once had. Grief is the only way I can describe the feelings when these thoughts began to surface. She might well have come to manage her illness and live with it for a long time, with many wonderful times ahead . . . but we were all changed by our changing of roles. I could see that I would struggle to let her care for me when her mental health had been under so much strain. But I had to let go of the idea we would go back to how things were.

This is a common scenario in many caring situations. Relationships that have been a certain way, sometimes for an entire lifetime, change drastically and it can be hard to accept those changes. Relationship changes can trigger very strong feelings of grief, anger and resentment. A person who relied very heavily on their partner for emotional support throughout their marriage may find themselves suddenly without that support as they become their carer. A parent who has been the rock-solid foundation of the family may struggle to be vulnerable and in need of support from their children. Becoming accustomed to an impairment or illness is an extremely difficult process for many people. It can often be hard to accept support and not everyone is grateful for the care they receive. Many carers give up paid work, change their living arrangements and rearrange their lives to provide support. That can leave some feeling resentful that so much has been asked of them, even if it was their choice to do so.

The grief of changing relationships

It can be difficult to speak about grief when the person we love is still alive. But our emotions as humans are rarely the tidy things we wish for them to be. I'm not sure that I would have been able to describe my feelings of grief as a teenager but as soon as my mother died I realised that's exactly what I'd been feeling for years. I couldn't admit before she died that I had been so hurt by her illness that I experienced grief. If my mother had known that, she would have been devastated. I didn't pretend that I found it easy but I was never able to be open with her about my feelings in case she blamed herself for it.

This is not an experience exclusive to those whose loved ones have mental illnesses. Progressive neurological conditions such as Huntington's, Alzheimer's and dementia, and motor nueron disease, to give a few examples, all lead to emotional and psychological changes in a person that can mean a relationship is irreversibly altered. The nature of all those diseases – that there are no known cures – also means that death is inevitable. Caring for someone with these disorders means a constant adaptation to their mental and physical decline which will only end in one way. While my autistic son might be more vulnerable to some co-occurring conditions such as epilepsy, right now there is no reason not to suppose that he will lead a long and reasonably healthy life. This is not the same for many carers, who may not know how much time they have, but do know that death is the inevitable end of their role supporting a loved one.

Emma Terranova was 14 when her parents sat her and her older sister Kelly down and told them that their mother Jenny had Huntington's disease (HD). Jenny had known for many years already but it had begun to be difficult to hide some of her symptoms. Her own mother had died before Emma was born, when Kelly was one and Jenny was 28, and the HD diagnosis was confirmed at the time of her death. Jenny was among the first generation of people to have access to the genetic test that would confirm if you were a carrier: Huntington's is hereditary, with a person carrying the gene having a 50% chance of passing it on to their children. It's a disease that until very recently has mostly been hidden; in the past, families often didn't even know relatives had died of the disease. Due to the nature of personality changes and mental health issues associated with it, people who had it were often sent to psychiatric hospitals and hidden away by their families; people did not understand the condition. It is a neurological condition with the symptoms typically beginning between 30 and 50 years old (although there is also a juvenile onset version which can start much earlier), and which damages the brain irreversibly. Symptoms typically include mood changes, depression, involuntary jerky movements, difficulty concentrating and memory problems. Eventually there are problems moving, swallowing, speaking and breathing. Death will typically occur around 15 to 20 years after the onset of symptoms.

When Emma found out about her mother's illness, Jenny had already been experiencing neurological changes that were making it hard for her to be rational and control her anger. She also had involuntary movements in one of her legs and in her fingers. Emma described her mother Jenny before HD as warm, loving and extremely affectionate. After her mother had disclosed the diagnosis, she very quickly became very depressed, often irrational and difficult to live with. Emma isn't sure whether that was a natural result of HD or if the full weight of the diagnosis had finally hit her once her daughters were aware of it. The uniquely difficult situation with Huntington's is that not only must children come to terms with their parent's inevitable deterioration, both mental and physical, but they too have a 50%

chance of facing the same fate themselves. In telling her daughters about her diagnosis, Jenny was also giving them the news that they and any children they might choose to have might be confronting a similar future.

With Kelly away at university, leaving two weeks after they found out about their mother's Huntington's, Emma began to depend more on herself as Jenny's mood swings increased. 'One day she would make me a bolognese and be cuddly and affectionate, the next she's throwing a pan at my head,' Emma explained to me when we spoke. Not really understanding the nature of the illness, Emma struggled to imagine it as anything other than her own fault. She became angry at her father's seemingly passive acceptance of her mother's behaviour. Looking back, she says that of course her father understood that it was HD that was making her behave as she did and that he knew there was no point fighting it or blaming her. As her mother deteriorated further, it became Emma's responsibility, with her dad, to do the cooking, washing and shopping. But it wasn't easy. Jenny was often convinced she could still do many things and, as she wasn't always able to make rational decisions, it became increasingly difficult to keep her safe.

Emma describes those years as a time of great loss. Her mother's personality had changed so much, she was now a young carer and she had to come to terms with the idea that she might too have the disease. At the same time she wasn't allowed to discuss this with anyone, hiding her mother's illness from everyone – including her paternal grandparents – because of the shame associated with the illness. Emma is not alone in this; many people with a parent with Huntington's are forbidden from speaking about it. Emma says this has only increased the problems they have faced as a family and it's the one thing she still feels angry at her parents for, even though she understands why they did it. The disease is not well understood by the general public, nor by medical professionals and social workers. Emma recalls taking her mother shopping as a teenager only to have strangers assume her mother was drunk, due to her jerky movements and angry outbursts. She says that if her mother had been elderly, people would have been more compassionate, understanding that it might have been dementia or Parkinson's. But a woman in her forties with a teenage daughter in tow receives nothing but derision and nasty comments. Before the illness, her mother had been extremely proud and would have been horrified to be looked down on as she so often was when they were out and about in those years. While her mother had become uninhibited due to the disease and didn't seem to be so affected by the difficulty they had in public, Emma felt all of it deeply.

It is 16 years since Emma learned of her mother's illness. Jenny is still living with Emma's dad and Emma lives a couple of miles away with her husband and her five-year-old daughter Rosa. Emma stayed close by for university and afterwards, remaining available to her parents when they needed her. She is a paramedic and splits her time between full-time shifts, supporting her mother, co-ordinating all her social care and medical administration and looking after her own family. Jenny's symptoms remained quite stable for many years. Although she was no longer able to drive or leave the house on her own, she was still able to attend to her own personal care and spend time alone in the house, with Emma calling periodically to check on her and popping around regularly. Around the time Emma became pregnant with Rosa, Jenny's symptoms increased quite suddenly. Emma's father came home one evening to find her sitting in the dark. He asked her why she didn't turn the lights on and she couldn't remember why. They also realised she was forgetting to drink anything and had lost the ability to plan arrangements for eating. She now needed help to eat, and choking was a serious risk. It became clear that she needed someone with her all the time. As Emma went on maternity leave, with her dad still working and her sister living too far away to come over regularly, it became her responsibility to support her mum every day until social services could help.

Emma recalls having a tiny baby Rosa asleep upstairs while she was in the kitchen with her mother, feeding her lunch. Rosa woke and began to cry just as Jenny began to choke. Emma managed to stop the choking but her mother was extremely distressed. With Rosa crying upstairs for a feed (she was breast-fed so solely reliant on Emma feeding her) and her mother crying and not safe to leave alone downstairs, Emma felt completely torn with the impossibility of it all. It's so hard to explain to people what that feels like, she told me, to not be able to reach your baby when they're crying. In the end it took a year and a formal complaint for social services to recognise Jenny's high needs. In that time Emma was diagnosed with post-natal depression and anxiety, and became so burned out that not long after returning to work, she had to be signed off sick. Emma's father also experienced a burnout, collapsing in front of their house. In the four years since then, Jenny is now using a wheelchair and dependent on carers for all her needs. Emma says ironically that as her needs have become higher, it's actually been easier to manage. Despite many dangerous falls, Jenny could not recognise her need for a mobility aid and refused a wheelchair for years, making it extremely difficult for Emma to take her out safely. The inability to recognise one's own needs is very common with Huntington's, which can add to the stress of supporting someone with the disease. The lack of understanding around the cognitive impairment with Huntington's meant that Jenny's behaviours could not be managed easily, and were completely unpredictable. In fact the reason the family waited a whole year for social-care support when her symptoms increased was because the social worker had no understanding at all of the disease and simply took Jenny's word for it when she said she could do everything on her own.

When we spoke, Emma said that her mother will hopefully be with them for another year or two. When I asked her how she feels about the future, she says she's scared. Her mother now spends a great deal of the day anxious and distressed, which is by far the most difficult thing for them all. At a certain point the disease will progress and she will struggle to swallow even more than she does now. In disorders like Huntington's, a feeding tube may be inserted into the stomach to ensure calorie intake remains high and to prevent dehydration. But the nature of her mother's extreme distress means it may not be safe to do that, as she might pull it out; Jenny also made an advance decision that she did not want a feeding tube. Over the years Emma and her sister Kelly have become very open about their family situation. Jenny agreed to them speaking about it publicly, even deciding to take part in a documentary that Kelly and a friend have filmed and will be releasing in 2020. She was able to see now that the shame around Huntington's only made their situation far more isolating than it would have been, and she supports her daughter's desire to see neurological conditions more widely recognised by both the public and medical professionals.

Among Emma's fears about how things will progress over the next couple of years is also a recognition that it will soon be time to reach the next stage of grief for her mother. A process that began the day her parents told them the news. Over the years, as she has adjusted to the changes in her relationship with her mother, she and her sister have also had the prospect of facing up to their own mortality. In her early twenties, Emma decided it was time to have the genetic test to see if she was positive. Due to the nature of the illness and the associated risk of suicide associated with a positive result, you must receive genetic counselling before a test is given. Emma had recently met her husband and had been very open with him about her mother's diagnosis. The results would influence whether they decided to have children or not. The day she received her results, she went straight to see her mother to tell her the good news that she didn't carry the gene. It was only a few years ago, when Kelly found herself unexpectedly pregnant, and with the potential of passing on the gene, that she too decided it was time she knew. Jenny was far less able to communicate by this stage but when she heard that Kelly was not a carrier either, tears ran down her face. Her daughters had a very different future ahead of them to the one that she and her own mother had experienced. Emma is sure that knowledge brought huge relief to her. When she asked Jenny how it felt, she said, *'euphoric.'*

Anticipatory grief

Something that is rarely spoken about in our society is anticipatory grief. Anna Lyons is an end-of-life doula. She supports people who are dying, along with their friends and family, before and often after the death. Anna believes that we need to get better at speaking about and being open about death. That dying is an important part of living and that death is a normal part of life. It's so important, she told me when we spoke, that we recognise anticipatory grief. It's normal for a dying person to experience it and it's normal for carers and loved ones to experience it too. Grief doesn't wait for death to occur. We can experience it well before death, as we imagine a future without our loved ones, and as we imagine the other losses we will go through before they die.

Anna works with her client, and their family and friends who are supporting them, to figure out what it is they need. She can act as an advocate, co-ordinating between the different services that person uses, as a central point, and can make referrals to services like palliative care. With family and friends, she says, it's often about preparing them and giving them the confidence to support their loved one themselves. We can all do it, Anna says, we just lack the confidence. Carers are often supporting someone for the first time and, though they are capable, they often may not realise it. It's about empowering them. Anna describes her job as helping to create a pyramid of care, with the person who is ill at the top, loved ones caring for them just below them, followed by another layer of support for the carers.

While it can be difficult to see someone you love experience so many losses as a condition progresses, it can have another side to it. Lucy and I grew up together on the same street. Her mother Rae was like a second mother to me, just as my mother Christine was to Lucy. We spent our childhoods racing between each other's homes within the tight-knit community of our quiet dead-end road. Rae was diagnosed with Alzheimer's aged 64, after experiencing symptoms for a while. That was 10 years ago and Rae, who is supported at home by Lucy's dad David, is reaching a more advanced stage of the illness now, requiring round-the-clock support. When I spoke to David, we talked about the changes Rae has been experiencing the past year. Up until quite recently the disease had been slow and steady, giving them both time to adjust to Rae's needs as they progressed. Now he is facing up to the fact that at some point in the near future he may not be able to support her in the same ways. He has a bit of help from paid carers for a few hours during the day and the kids also help him out, but David has been doing the vast majority of Rae's care. Rae can become very distressed when anyone else supports her for more than a few hours, even when it's one of her three children, so David has been putting off any increased help. But Lucy and her siblings worry about their dad's health and want to make sure he doesn't push himself so hard that they lose him too. While they want to do all they can to minimise Rae's distress as the disease progresses, they want their dad to lead as long and healthy a life as possible after their mum's death.

I asked David if he thinks much about the future, once Rae has died and he is no longer a carer. He says that his children's confidence that he will have a life afterwards has had a positive effect. He has grandchildren to spend time with, a house and garden to tend to and old friends with whom he doesn't get to socialise as often as he would like. He knows he will feel very low for a time but he's hoping that with so much to live for, he will make the most of his time when he is no longer a full-time carer. David is a recently retired GP and certainly no stranger to illness and death, but says that his experience as a carer has been extremely eye-opening. In all his years a GP, he never really paid that much attention to the unpaid carers who were supporting his patients at home. It's unimaginable really, he tells me. You can describe what it's like to people, but no one can really understand what it's like to support someone in this way until you go through it. 'I wish I had known,' he tells me.

Rae will shortly be going for some respite care for three weeks. David has had this available to him for a while and has not been able to bring himself to access it. Rae's needs are complex, as she is now also very visually impaired. But with an operation on his hand becoming necessary, it has given David the push he needed. After the operation he won't be able to drive, carry things or do anything with that hand for at least a week, making caring for Rae impossible. If he leaves the operation any longer, the damage to his hand may not be reversible. Without a solid reason such as this, it's been easy to ignore his own needs for the past couple of years and avoid getting more help, despite his kids asking him to do so. He knows that not everyone would have been able to provide the kind of support that he has been able to with Rae. He admits it's been very hard but he's still extremely glad he has been able to do it. It has been best for both Rae and himself. He's been reluctant to admit that it can't necessarily continue indefinitely, but he's grateful to have been able to do it for as long as he has.

Anna Lyons has supported many carers through the loss of a loved one. After years of sometimes intense levels of care supporting a child, partner or parent, it becomes the central point on which your whole life pivots. When that disappears, it can leave a cavernous void. As difficult as supporting someone through illness can be, it is a strong reason to get out of bed every morning. If someone is relying on you, it just has to be done. When that is gone, it can be very hard to cope with the sudden lack of purpose. Anna says she sees it especially in older married couples. A carer is often extremely self-sufficient, rarely asking for help, and because of their caring responsibilities may have slowly retreated from much of their former social contact, spending days at a time with no one but their spouse whom they are supporting. When that person dies, the isolation can be intense.

As Anna says, we are not good as a society at talking about both death and caring. Death as a topic is still deeply uncomfortable for people, despite it being the only inevitable part of life. And caring, both paid and unpaid, is so looked down on that many people don't bring it up in conversation. In order to support each other through difficult times, we must start talking about it, she tells me. Death is after all a part of life. If we are to support someone to live the best life they can, for as long as possible, conversations about death are a vital part of that.

Mitzi and her father Maurice talk very openly about his death. They don't know how long it will be but with a diagnosis of motor neuron disease, it is inevitable. Maurice lives in his own apartment with government-provided carers coming in to see him every morning. He spends his days alone, still able to transfer between his hospital bed and electric wheelchair, still able to control the chair himself, retaining a little independence. Each evening one of his daughters comes over to cook dinner and spend time with him. Mitzi is his primary carer, co-ordinates all his medical and social care admin and takes him to all his appointments.

Unlike everyone I have spoken to in a similar situation, Maurice, who lives in Montreal, has access to medically assisted dying and has decided at some point he may choose when the end of his life will be. I asked Mitzi how she and her sisters feel about the decision. She told me that it made her dad feel far more relaxed about his future, knowing that he is in control. That alone is something to be grateful for and so she's glad for his sake that it's available to him. She said, though, that she does have to remind him that she supports whatever decision he makes. That she will continue supporting him till the end no matter when or how that might be. She doesn't want him to think of anything but what he wants when it comes to the end of his life.

Knowing death is coming

Mitzi is no stranger to grief. Her mother died of cancer 10 years ago when she was 22 years old. She is already anticipating the loss of her dad, feeling the familiarity of grief as the disease progresses. His diagnosis was long and drawn out. He was initially misdiagnosed and even went through unnecessary chemotherapy treatment as a result. When the diagnosis finally came, they were devastated: motor neuron disease, or ALS as it is known in Canada, has no cure. Earlier this year, she began a blog about her experiences as a caregiver to help her process her thoughts and to connect with others in similar circumstances. She writes about the firsts and lasts that she and her dad go through together. The first time she has to do his buttons for him, the first time she has to cut his food, the first time she wrote her own birthday card. The lasts are realised much later – in retrospect – and already she feels like they are a long time ago. The last time he drove her in a car, the last time he made an important phone call alone, the last time he cooked for himself. It's a slow and long process of letting go for them both, she tells me. But in all the changes in their relationship, she still feels cared for by him. He sends her texts during the day, still has a sense of humour and sends her home with lots of food. She says remembering this and remembering that even though she is his carer she will always be his daughter first, has helped ease the feelings of grief.

Just as the person being supported may experience a long series of losses, perhaps in mobility, cognition or communication, being a carer can mean experiencing losses too. As Mitzi describes, the changes that have occurred in her father have affected her and the relationship they have. Each one can take time to adjust to. Those smaller losses can feel devastating. A painful letting go of a person and the relationship you had with them bit by bit. Recognising those feelings as a part of the grieving process is important.

Caring for someone can also have a knock-on effect on other relationships too. When you are busy supporting someone, friendships can fall by the wayside, time with children may have to be cut short, your spouse may see much less of you. It can at times be all-encompassing which can lead to sadness, resentment and isolation. A number of people told me that when a parent needed intense levels of care, not only did they provide a lot of that support, but so did their other parent. It felt like they had lost both parents at once. One who was dying, and the other busy caring for the dying.

Kieran Rose (see Chapter 3, page 82) spent the last few years of his father's life supporting him through emphysema and a number of other chronic illnesses. Like Kieran, his father was autistic, although remained undiagnosed. He was living around the corner from Kieran and his family, and as his needs increased, Kieran found some days he was spending up to 20 hours with him. With three young children at home, the situation wasn't sustainable. Like so many, his father struggled accepting support from paid carers. He had been such a strongly independent man throughout his life and the only way he coped with everything was to control his surroundings and do things exactly as they suited him. Kieran tried to explain this to the paid carers who had started to help support his father at home, but he said you could practically see the eye rolls when he mentioned autism. They told him he was making a fuss, that his father was old, nothing more. They continually ignored Kieran's requests for them to adapt the way they approached his care needs. Eventually Kieran's father conceded that he needed some support, although the process would have been less traumatic for everyone if his needs had been better understood by social services.

Despite how difficult that time was, juggling his father's needs and those of his three children, Kieran is grateful for the experience. His father had been a workaholic all his life, and when he wasn't working he was drinking. Kieran can look back now and see how this had happened. It was how he coped with masking his autistic tendencies. Becoming dependent on Kieran changed things significantly for the whole family. He couldn't escape into work any more and, with his health as it was, he could no longer drink. In those last few years he spent more time with Kieran than he had in his entire life. Despite the difficulties, they became closer than they had ever been. Over at Kieran's house he would sit and watch films with the children, who would climb onto his lap. It was something Kieran had never experienced as a child and he was amazed to see a relationship grow between his children and their grandfather.

Kieran's father died of heart failure at his home, just as Kieran was popping in to check on him one afternoon. Although they were an extremely intense few years, he wouldn't change them for a moment.

This kind of positive transformation of a relationship between a carer and someone who is ill is not always going to be possible. Relationships shift and change and not always for the better. It's sometimes hard for people to accept support, or to give so much of it, and that tension can fracture relationships. Carers often find that no matter what is expected of them, no matter what the state of the relationship, they cannot walk away. This can leave a carer feeling intense resentment towards the person they care for. Others, like Kieran, find the relationship deepens and becomes richer than at any other point in their lives and even though it can be extremely hard, it can also be deeply rewarding.

Saying goodbye

The night before my mother's funeral, we all gathered as a family at the funeral home for the viewing. The only people in my life who had died up until this point were my great-grandmother and a dear friend of my parents who had died in his early forties. I had never been to a funeral before. I didn't know how I felt about seeing my mother's body. My mother's family are Catholic and they insisted it was important, so I took their word for it. My brothers and I stood in the main chapel with our dad. It had taken almost a week for us all to get back to Melbourne. Pip had been travelling around Queensland without a mobile phone, Ash was living in the US, Dad had been in Canada and I had been in London. It was my mother's two sisters who had been called to the hospital after my mum had been found by a close friend. My aunts had been the ones to make the call to shut off her life support when it became clear there was nothing else to be done. They had been able to say their goodbyes then, but my brothers and I had yet to see her. When we went into the smaller chapel where she lay in an open coffin, I was glad not to be alone. She seemed so tiny and frail. She wore the dress she bought for her 40th birthday celebration. It was vintage lace, Edwardian in style with a high neck, and though the funeral home had done an excellent job, I could make out the marks around her neck that gave away how she died. It was suddenly so real. The coldness of her skin as I touched her hand and gave her a rosary. She looked so at peace but she was not sleeping. I let out a huge sigh. I suddenly understood why my aunts had insisted we see her. This was not an imagined scenario I had worried myself into inventing. She really was dead.

Back in the larger chapel we sat and talked as other family members went to see her. We found ourselves telling stories and laughed as Dad recounted the tale of winning my mother over from her ex-fiancé in an argument that almost ended in a fist fight. Everyone took turns, as we all eagerly waited to hear more stories from before we were born. My mother as a child, as a teenager, as a young wife. My mother, the middle sister and the daddy's girl, who had lost her father very suddenly when she was the exact age I was then. I realised I felt far less afraid, and when everyone else had seen her, I decided to go back in alone. When I approached her I took her hand properly this time. I looked at her and told her I was so proud of her. That I knew how hard she had tried to stay with us. That I was so glad she hadn't died when I was 14. That I wish her care had been better, that I could have done more to stop her suffering. That she was the most wonderful mother I could have asked for. No one could have better prepared me for her illness and death than she had, with her insightfulness, her love and kind-heartedness.

The funeral was held in my mother's childhood church, on the road she grew up in. It was packed to the rafters, although I couldn't tell you who was there. It was February and baking hot. My best friend Marisa and I had spent an entire day searching shops for a black outfit to wear, which was hard in the midst of late-summer sales. I found myself taking dark pleasure in telling shop assistants that I needed an outfit for my mother's funeral and watching them squirm. Marisa and I laughed about it in the car afterwards, a much-needed relief after funeral plans, will-reading and decisions to be made. After the long service was over, I followed Mum's coffin out of the church. As everyone started to come out behind us, I could barely take in the blur of familiar faces, many of whom I hadn't seen for years. But there was one face that stood out to me in particular. I saw my school housemistress quietly coming out of the service alone. I hadn't seen her since I had left school four years earlier. A new term had not long started and we were almost two hours' drive from my old school. I didn't know how she had known my mother had died, or how she had managed to get away for the day to come to the funeral. In that moment I had a sudden overwhelming urge to tell her how much the school had meant to me when Mum was too ill to look after me. That I would never forget all they did to support me and encourage me. But I choked and sobbed and no words came out.

I wondered if I would be afraid to get back on the plane. That after the house was packed up, all my mother's possessions split between the three of us and my portion shipped off to storage, that I wouldn't be able to leave. But after two weeks, I found myself looking forward to returning to London. I had a new job and new flatmates waiting. A whole new life, one where I wouldn't constantly be waiting for phone calls that would turn my world upside-down. I was no longer responsible for anyone but myself. A strange and untethering feeling after years of worry. Although I had already moved across the world, I had fully expected to be on the end of the phone often, fielding panicked phone calls, organising trips back. But a tie had been cut. Not just between my mother and me, but with my home-town too. Without her I no longer had a family home or a central point. It was strange and unsettling feeling. More like free-falling than freedom. My body almost tingled with the sensations of being alive. Perhaps it was the contrast of my mother's cold body, but mine now felt more alive than it ever had. I could feel pain and excitement and fear and anxiety, while my mother could feel nothing at all. I almost revelled in it because this is what it meant to love and be alive. I reminded myself that I had experienced just about the worst thing that can happen. There was nothing to be afraid of now.

I was wrong, of course. 15 years later, with a failing marriage and a child I didn't know how to support, the scar left by her death felt like it was being ripped open again. The grief resurfaced stronger than ever. I wept for her and raged at the injustice that she wasn't here when I needed her most. She would have adored Arthur. I could almost picture her in my mind playing with him and calming him when he was upset. He would have gained so much from her being in his life. I would try and imagine what it would be like having a mother to call after years of not having her. Memories of her sleeping through afternoons reared up. Of her attempting to get into the car drunk. Of long hospital stays and arguments over whether I was doing enough to help her. Things I hadn't thought about for years. I wasn't just feeling grief over her death but for the years beforehand when I had been slowly letting her go. I imagined my own children having to do the same for me and it made me feel physically sick.

When I visited Melbourne for the first time after my son's diagnosis it was alone and for my best friend Marisa's wedding. The night before the wedding I sat with her mum Shirley and told her everything that had been happening over the previous couple of years. Shirley is a retired GP and the mother of five children. Marisa is her eldest, and her second daughter Yasmin was born with Down's syndrome. As I explained the difficulties Arthur was having, the lack of support and the learning I was doing to help meet his needs, she smiled and reminded me of the most important thing I needed to remember as a mother. 'You think when your child is born with a disability that it's the end of the world. But it really isn't.' Yasmin had died suddenly and unexpectedly when she was 13. I thought in that moment how much Shirley would give to still be supporting Yasmin, 20 years on. Of how she expected that Yasmin would always need her, more than her other children, but that she was gone. It was exactly the reminder I needed to focus on all the things I did have. When I returned to London a few days later about to face life as a single parent, it was with a renewed energy for the challenges life had thrown my way and a deep sense of gratitude that I had the chance to experience life with Arthur, challenges and all.

CHAPTER 6

Self-Care

'Taking care of yourself doesn't mean me first; it means me too.'[57]

L.R. Knost, author

Suzy Reading was nine months pregnant the night she accompanied her father to hospital. He had been unwell for many months, experiencing unusual symptoms that no one could identify the cause of. It became clear as the doctors saved her father's life that night that he would not be returning home or returning to his former state of good health. His diagnosis of a rare form of motor neuron disease wouldn't come until after his death 15 months later. During this time Suzy gave birth to her first child Charlotte, helped her mother support her father in hospital and then move him to a care facility. She also supported her mother through a hospital stay for cellulitis, spending her days travelling from the hospital her father lay in to the one her mother was in the other side of Sydney, all while caring for a colicky newborn who wouldn't sleep for more than an hour or two at a time. Suzy had a career as a wellness coach, with a psychology degree and years of experience helping women to look after themselves through fitness and yoga. Yet, for the first time, she felt so depleted and drained that she couldn't even pull her yoga mat out.

It was a post-natal counsellor who helped support Suzy to make the first few changes she needed to in order to get through this period of irreversible change. What she came to realise over time was that all the tips and tricks she had relied on in the past simply weren't fit for purpose any more. When once she would meditate for 20 minutes, have a run on the beach, time out and about seeing friends and getting eight hours of sleep a night, suddenly none of this was possible. The very thought of trying to squeeze in even one of those things was overwhelming. As someone who had thought she knew how to look after herself, Suzy felt completely lost.

Self-care has become a bit of a buzz word, bandied about in articles about hot baths and taking time out. And it would be easy to get cynical about the term. Its use by people who have little responsibility for anyone but themselves could easily make it seem like individualism taken to its extreme. Feminist writer Laurie Penny wrote in 2016 of the wellness trend of which self-care is a part, that it perpetuates the idea that 'if you are miserable or angry because your life is a constant struggle against privation or prejudice, the problem is always and only with you. Society is not mad, or messed up: you are.'[58] In writing about self-care in this book, I want to make it perfectly clear it is in no way a replacement for the collective responsibility society needs to take in supporting those of us who are unpaid family carers. We cannot expect to make up for a lack of respite and for the energy we expend fighting for basic services for our loved ones by practising a bit of yoga.

This chapter is not intended to add to anyone's already insurmountable to-do list or to put responsibility for our own wellbeing on our already overloaded selves. It is simply here to remind us that we are also worth standing up for and being cared for. In the words of black activist and writer Audre Lorde, who wrote in her essay *A Burst Of Light* about living with cancer: 'Caring for myself is not self-indulgence, it is self-preservation, and that is an act of political warfare.'[59] Carers are not just carers. Carers are also more likely to be women, more likely to be living in poverty and under- or unemployed. They're more likely to have poor mental health or physical health. Carers may also be disabled themselves and part of other marginalised communities such as being of colour or LGBQT+. When self-care is considered in the context of those who put the needs of others so often before their own, it can be nothing short of life saving. What carers need most is a set of non-negotiables, things that they know will keep them going through difficult times.

Read any of the recommendations for self-care and most may seem ridiculously out of reach. Articles on the importance of sleep can leave us feeling anxious about the damage being done daily when our sleep patterns feel completely out of our control, dictated by the needs of another person. Preparing healthy meals can seem impossible between the juggle of work and supporting someone else's care needs. Getting to an exercise class? Forget it. But is it *all* impossible? It can feel that way. And sometimes we get in our own way, not prioritising what is essential. If we don't learn to look after ourselves, the consequences can be catastrophic for us and for those we care for.

Caregiver burnout is a phenomenon now widely recognised by medical professionals. Symptoms can range from low mood, feeling helpless, physical exhaustion, stress-related illness such as high blood pressure, rage, overreacting, insomnia, substance abuse and anxiety. Amongst the most distressing symptoms are self-harm, suicidal thoughts and thoughts of harming the person you are caring for. In a report for Carers UK, those caring for a family member for more than 50 hours a week felt the worst effects, with 25% reporting they had either bad or very bad physical health, and 29% reporting bad or very bad mental health.[60] We cannot always control the levels of support we receive from social care services, or support from other family members, but we should never underestimate the need for our own health and wellbeing to be equal to those of the person we are supporting.

What exactly is self-care? It is a set of skills and practices that we use regularly in order to stay physically, mentally and emotionally healthy. When Suzy Reading found herself lost in her new role caring for a newborn and her father at the same time, she said it took her time to realise that what she now needed as a carer was a completely *different* set of tools. Ones that were much more manageable, that didn't add to her already overwhelmed mind and exhausted body. Over time things changed, and Suzy developed ways of coping, adding tools to her kit and beginning to feel like herself again. A couple of years after the death of her father, with a toddler and a second baby, Suzy and her husband received the news that his father was extremely unwell and so the whole family moved across the world to the UK to support him in his last few months of life. This time Suzy had an array of skills to keep herself afloat and at no point – despite the extreme difficulties – did she experience the same level of exhaustion and overwhelm as she had during her first experience as a caregiver and new parent. She is certain this was because she had a much broader range of coping skills that she was now well accustomed to using. She was able to pick and choose things that were manageable to her in those difficult moments. Suzy wrote about her experiences and the skills and practices she discovered in her book *The Self-Care Revolution*.

During my teenage years my mother and I spent hours talking about the things that led her to such a state of poor mental health. She had been a classic martyr mother and it was only after periods of being completely unable to look after us had she realised just how damaging 'doing it all' had been. There were many reasons for my mum's mental health decline, much of which were out of her control. But we talked about the things she regretted, the things within her control that she could have approached differently. There were times when she begged me to learn from her mistake of thinking that every other person in our family should come before herself. It is easy as a parent or caregiver to put the acute and often urgent needs of another person in front of you. There will be times when it is absolutely necessary, but we have a duty of care to ourselves to ensure that when the urgency has passed, we meet our own needs as well. Perhaps my mother's life would have looked different had she learned much earlier to consider her own needs alongside ours. In the end, her suffering meant we all suffered. Not taking better care of herself was a regret she held the rest of her life.

My mother was not to blame for this. We live in a patriarchal society where caregivers of all kinds, traditionally and predominantly women, are socialised to put the needs of others before themselves. We are praised for doing so and we are chastised and told we are selfish if we dare to put our own needs first. Inequality in caregiving may be shrinking but it still remains that women do the bulk of the unpaid work. Currently women make up 57% of carers in the UK but there are indications that they do a greater amount of the care. As mentioned in the Introduction, in families with a disabled child, for instance, 84% of mothers do no paid work compared to 39% of mothers of non-disabled children. Only 3% of us with disabled kids work full time.[61] I think it is a fair assessment to suggest that it is mothers who are taking on the majority of care for disabled children. An Office for National Statistics (ONS) time survey study from 2016 shows that women on average still do 60% more unpaid work in households. That means that men do an average of 16 hours of unpaid labour per week while women do 26 hours.[62]

In their book *Burnout*, Emily and Amelia Nagoski describe what they have coined Human Giver Syndrome. It is based on the work of philosopher Kate Manne's theory of 'Human Beings' and 'Human Givers', which asserts that some humans have the moral obligation to *be* their whole humanity while others have the obligation to *give* their whole humanity. They describe Human Giver Syndrome as believing you have a moral obligation to prioritise being 'pretty, happy, calm, generous and attentive to the needs of others, above anything else.'[63] Nothing could more perfectly describe many of the carers I have come to know over the years. My mother was certainly a casualty of this syndrome.

This accounts for a lot of the guilt that we feel as primary carers, as we attempt to carve out more time for ourselves. Even just becoming aware of how our society thrives on a certain section of us giving our all and taking nothing for ourselves, goes some way to help alleviate the guilt that many carers feel when trying to prioritise their own needs. Suzy Reading told me that guilt is one of the major reasons why people claim they can't possibly consider more self-care. She finds helping them to reframe self-care as something that helps facilitate the other roles in their life is a good way around this. If a carer understands what the consequences of being unable to support their loved one may be, that can act as motivation to make their own health needs a priority. Listening to Suzy describe how some caregivers are only able to look after themselves if they see that it helps their loved ones makes me feel terribly sad. But however we get there, get there we must. We cannot function in long-term caring situations if we do not rest and take care of ourselves, especially when we are dealing with high levels of stress in our roles as carers. We are worthy of a little time and priority spent on ourselves and our own health.

Rest

Simply getting enough rest can be a huge challenge for carers who are living with and caring for a family member who needs them much of the day and night. Suzy is not alone in her experience caring for a newborn who barely slept as well as helping support her father throughout the day. She is a part of what's referred to as the 'sandwich generation', people who have both children or grandchildren and parents to care for simultaneously.

If a night of unbroken sleep is inaccessible, the priority needs to become rest. Suzy was frazzled and exhausted when a post-natal counsellor suggested that she rest in the tiny moments her daughter would sleep during the day. She had been avoiding going to bed to try to sleep, because each time she did she would be resentful and upset when her baby would inevitably wake after just 20 minutes. Getting some sleep during those brief times became too pressure-filled. When the counsellor suggested she reclaim a practice she used to find nourishing, she rolled out her yoga mat and lay in a restorative pose, swaddled in blankets, and just rested. Sometimes she fell asleep but she didn't have to. It was the rest that was important and it was completely free from pressure. After a very short time of diligently resting whenever the baby slept, Suzy felt some energy returning to her body, and her mind became a little less foggy.

There is nothing more infuriating then being told to get more sleep when more sleep is inaccessible. But viewing it as rest can really help make it more achievable. We can rest in small moments throughout the day; we don't need to be in bed to do it. Resting has an accumulative effect, which means those grabbed moments here and there really do add up. Before she had tried resting on her yoga mat, Suzy had been using her baby's short naps to lie on the sofa and watch daytime soaps on TV. She said she had to first acknowledge that this was not helping her before she could find a better way. It really worked. Regaining some energy was the first of many important steps she took towards feeling like her whole self again.

Suzy recommends firstly prioritising sleep, but there are going to be times in our lives when that's just not in our control, so rest and relaxation need to be our next priority. And if there isn't time even to be still? You work with your breath. As Suzy says: 'Sleep, rest, relaxation and breathing all stimulate the parasympathetic nervous system. If you can't sleep, then rest, if there is no time to rest, then work with your breath. There is always a way.'

Breath

It doesn't have to be fancy. Suzy recommends simply breathing in, noticing the moment after we inhale, breathing out and then noticing that moment after. Even 30 to 60 seconds can be enough to calm the nervous system of stress hormones. Peppered throughout the day, it can be a huge help to our exhausted bodies and minds. Suzy refers to these moments as micro moments of self-care, and they are genuinely accessible to all of us. We have to breathe anyway, so we may as well use our breath in an effective, expansive way. She reminded me that it's important not to get worried about doing it right or wrong. It's not about striving. Again, that just adds too much pressure. It's simply remembering to take deep breaths at different times throughout the day. We can piggy-back the habit of breathing onto other activities we might already be doing, and use those activities as a trigger to remember to breathe. Like boiling the kettle, putting on our shoes or stopping at a red light.

Sleep

We still need sleep and we need to be creative about how we get it. Like many aspects of life as a carer, how we get sleep might look a lot different to how other people do it, and that's ok. Arthur goes to sleep around 9pm each night, and about once or twice a week he starts his day at 2am. Occasionally, in a bad patch, it may be up to three times a week. I do everything I can to promote good sleep for Arthur and myself but sometimes it's beyond my control.

Over the past 10 years, working freelance has been crucial for me getting enough rest. Having control over my time means I'm less likely to panic in the night when it becomes clear that Arthur is awake and will not be going back to sleep. I might grumble and be annoyed that I need to use precious work hours to have a nap, but that grumbling is usually caused by exhaustion. Once the kids are at school, if I am working from home that day, I have a sleep before I start work. If I'm struggling to switch off, my mind whirring with deadlines and to-do lists and how little time until the school day is over, I put on one of my meditation or hypno-therapy apps and listen with the intention of resting – which usually leads to a sleep.

There are days that I am with clients and I have no choice but to power through. Other days when it's a weekend or school holidays and I have the kids with me, I can't sleep. On those days I rest and make a mental note to catch up on sleep when I can.

Sometimes that might not be till the next weekend that my kids are with their dad. But extra sleep must happen at some point.

Mary Susan McConnell (see Chapter 4, page 93), whose daughter Abiella has had plenty of phases of poor sleep over the years, has come up with some ingenious solutions. Abiella, who has cerebral palsy and epilepsy, takes lots of medications and they sometimes cause sleep issues out of the blue. It can take a while for medications to be carefully adjusted, so as to improve her sleep but not disrupt the primary reason for the medication. These adjustments can take months. Added to that, exhaustion is a trigger for her seizures. One very late night not being able to fall asleep means Mary Susan has to allow her to have a lie-in in the morning, so she's not too tired. But then Abiella struggles to fall asleep the following night because she slept late. It's a vicious cycle. Mary Susan's husband Sean is a professional musician and spends a lot of time touring and so she is often Abiella's sole carer while he's away.

Aside from keeping her schedule as flexible as possible – completing her post-graduate degree from home, for instance – so she can sleep during the day if Abiella is also sleeping, Mary Susan decided to do something more radical occasionally. A handful of times during the year, before or after Sean is off on a tour, she checks in to a local hotel and doesn't leave it for 48 hours. She told me she only has a few criteria. It needs to be pretty cheap, have a balcony so she can sit outside, and access to some decent food. For 48 hours, she sleeps, reads, eats, enjoys a beer on the balcony, and when Abiella is at school, her husband Sean comes to meet her for a lunch date.

This is not a solution open to all. Mary Susan acknowledges that not everyone has the money or a partner or someone else confident enough to care for their loved one overnight, but she thinks often people don't do it because it either never occurs to them or they feel too guilty to try. It might take some planning to get another person ready to care for your parent, partner or child, but if the possibility is there, the hard work is absolutely worth it. We may need to beg for help, or pay for help if necessary, in order to get some much-needed rest (more on that in the Chapter 8). Mary Susan told me that knowing that a couple of days all to herself is coming up makes weeks of poor sleep much more bearable. I feel the same about the weekends that my children spend with their father.

Sleep is vital to our survival. Chronic sleep deprivation has a whole host of negative effects on our bodies and minds. In Matthew Walker's book, *Why We Sleep*, he describes the well-documented effects. 'Routinely sleeping less than six or seven hours a night demolishes your immune system, more than doubling your risk of cancer. Insufficient sleep is a key lifestyle factor in determining whether or not you will get Alzheimer's disease. Inadequate sleep, even moderate reductions for just one week, disrupts blood sugar so profoundly that you would be classified as pre-diabetic. Short sleeping increases the likelihood of your coronary arteries becoming blocked and brittle, setting you on a path towards cardiovascular disease, stroke and congestive heart failure.'[64] It is terrifying to be confronted with information like this when we are in a situation where we cannot get eight hours of uninterrupted sleep opportunity each night. But it's important to understand the risks of sleep deprivation in order to give ourselves fuel to fight for the sleep we need to carry out our caring duties, as well as simply live our lives.

If you cannot give yourself permission to rest for *yourself*, then you must do it for the person you care for. For Claire Kotecha (see Chapter 2, page 61) that meant taking social services to court to fight for night nurses to support her son. For others it may mean training another family member to support the person they care for and staying with a friend or going to a hotel occasionally.

Dealing with the stress in our bodies

Sleep and rest might be the first place to start to combat carer stress, but it doesn't end there. Emily and Amelia Nagoski explain in their book *Burnout*[65] that while there are times in our life when we cannot control the stressors, we must deal with the effects of stress itself. When Suzy first visited the GP to ask for help in the early days of caring for both her newborn and her father, she was told her options were to minimise stress or take antidepressants. The idea that we can just 'minimise stress' as caregivers is insulting and laughable. What Suzy could do, however, was deal with the stress in her body. She was able to start doing that after she had begun to regain some of her energy from her yoga mat rests.

As Emily and Amelia Nagoski point out in their book, it's important for us to distinguish the *stress* from the *stressor*. We may not always have control over the *stressor*. Sleepless nights, fighting for services, supporting a loved one through chronic pain or distress, are the stressors that create *stress* which accumulates in our bodies. Stress is the neurological and physiological response in our body to these stressors. When we are faced with a stressor our bodies respond in a way that makes it possible for us to protect us from the threat: also known as fight, flight or freeze. Whether it's a physical threat or a psychological one, our body reacts in the same way. Our heart rate increases, our blood pressure goes up, we release endorphins, our digestion slows down and so do other functions which are not necessary in the face of a perceived threat. This biological response affects our entire body and its function is to keep us alive. But as humans we are not built to live in a constant state of threat. 'If we get stuck there, the physiological responses intended to save us can instead slowly kill us,' is how the Nogoskis put it. We need to complete the stress cycle that has been activated in our bodies, and just telling ourselves that the threat is over doesn't do that.

In their book, the Nogoskis use the example of an early human running away from a wild animal. This is the situation the stress response has evolved to deal with. We perceive the threat and our body automatically makes changes to our physiology which in turn make it possible for us to run as fast as we possibly can. Once we've outrun the threat we are surrounded by our fellow villagers who hug us and remind us we are safe. The stress cycle is complete and our body can return to its relaxed physiological state. Faced with modern-day stressors, our bodies react in the same way but it's often not appropriate to run or physically defend ourselves. We deal with the stressor in front of us, for instance remaining calm and polite in a meeting in which you are arguing for services your loved one needs. But simply telling ourselves afterwards that the threat is over does not automatically reduce the raised blood pressure and the elevated hormones that are surging through our bodies. So we need to give our bodies the tools to complete the stress response cycle.

Movement

It was no surprise to me to hear from many other carers that one of their most important non-negotiables for themselves as a carer is the need to break a sweat. Every day. Moving our bodies is the most effective and efficient way to signal that a threat is over. Whether these carers have been conscious of completing their stress cycles or not, one thing is clear: movement is effective.

Jess Wilson, whose teenage daughter Brooke is autistic and has epilepsy (see Chapter 3, page 74), discovered Boot Camp a few years ago. Like many carers supporting a loved one with epilepsy, the stress that can accumulate from the hyper-vigilance required to keep a person who experiences seizures safe, can be acute. Constant hyper-vigilance may be something we are hardly even aware of; often we become so accustomed to it. Brooke started having severe tonic-clonic seizures in her early teens. Even with medication for a long time Brooke was having a life-threatening seizure at least once every six weeks. Jess said that although that doesn't sound like a lot, the problem is you are constantly watching and waiting for them to happen. She would drive Brooke to and from school each day in the car, anxious about Brooke seizing while they were driving, and fearful she wouldn't be able to get her safely out of the car. At home Brooke can no longer be left alone for a second and the family have taken to saying 'eyes' (on Brooke) out loud to whoever is present if they need to leave the room. Brooke's current medication is working well and she hasn't had a big seizure for nine months now. But Jess says she still finds it impossible to relax, as any number of factors could easily render an epilepsy drug ineffective again.

Jess said the discovery that rigorous exercise is such an effective way of dealing with her anxiety was transformative. She now knows that she must break a sweat for at least 20 minutes a day in order to counteract the stress that builds up. Before this she had been walking a lot and although she said that helped a bit, really getting an aerobic workout like the kind she gets at Boot Camp has made a huge difference. Our stress responses are physiological and so dealing with the stress by using our bodies – just as you would running away from a wild animal – is a great way to tell our bodies that we are now safe and the stress cycle can finish.

About a year ago, I started running. I had never imagined that I would enjoy running, but was tempted to try it after reading about the mental and physiological benefits. Add to that the fact it was free and completely flexible, I thought it was worth a try. I was surprised to find that I absolutely love it. In the South London neighbourhood where I live, we have lots of green spaces where I can run, see views across London and expanses of sky, watch the seasons change and be back at my desk in no time, feeling stronger and less stressed. And it can all be achieved by going outside my front door for 30 minutes. All I needed to get started was a £40 pair of running shoes and a free Couch to 5K running app.

While exercise and movement is one of the best ways to complete the stress cycle, it isn't the only way. Vigorous movement may be inaccessible to many people because of disability, illness or injury. Getting outside or getting to a class or the gym may be more than we can manage. Maybe the only chance you have to get outside alone is in the evening when it's dark and it doesn't feel safe for you. It might be effective but sometimes it's just not possible, especially when we are depleted of energy. But there are other ways to signal to our bodies that we are no longer under threat, and can relax.

Creative expression

Mary Susan lives on a rural property outside of Nashville, Tennessee. With the abundance of space they have, she has been able to convert one of their sheds into a pottery studio. For her 30th birthday, her husband Sean found her a potter's wheel on eBay and helped to set up the studio. She goes through busy periods, especially when Abiella isn't sleeping well, Sean is on tour, or while working on her doctoral degree, and she doesn't see a huge amount of the inside of that studio. But as soon as things calm down a little and she has more support, she makes it a priority to spent lots of time in there throwing some pots. She says that it's a combination of some time alone and the pleasure of creating something, with the sensory experience of touching the clay itself, which brings her a sense of calm and joy. Creative expression can be a great way to mitigate some of the effects of stress on our body. As with everything in Mary Susan's life, she says the key is to be flexible. Sometimes she doesn't make it into the studio for a while and that's ok. Other examples that carers gave me of creative expression that helped to reduce their stress were singing, playing piano and painting.

Touch

Hugging can also have a beneficial effect on the body. A 20-second hug can be an excellent way of signalling to our bodies that there is no threat and we can relax. Research shows that it can lower blood pressure and increase levels of oxytocin.[66] If no one else is around to touch, even our own touch can be an effective way of relaxing our bodies. Suzy Reading recommends getting some scented hand cream and taking 30–60 seconds to rub the lotion on to our hands. It sounds tiny, but the combination of a pleasant smell, taking a moment to stop and breathe it in, and the touch of our own hands, can be extremely effective.

Micro moments of calm

It is so easy to get caught up in the idea that self-care must be about grand gestures, expensive massages or classes, or long luxurious baths. Those things can be lovely but they aren't necessary and are often inaccessible. In her work supporting many new mothers, as well as mothers with disabled children, Suzy has found the most important thing is that we have lots of tools at our disposal, use them in tiny moments throughout the day and keep changing and evolving them, so that they stay fresh. For her it's about creating nourishing rituals around things we are doing anyway. We have to get dressed, so why not choose to wear something that has a texture that we love? She likes to have her clients ask themselves, 'How can I imbue everyday actions and activities with more tenderness, care and presence?' Everyone's list of self-care tools is going to look different. But one thing is certain, they do not have to be expensive, time-consuming or take a lot of energy. There are so many possibilities when it comes to self-care, so here are just a few more common and easy-to-access skills and tools that many people find useful.

Laughing, especially with other people, can be hugely beneficial to our bodies and minds. Laughter can relax tension in our muscles, release oxytocin, boost our immune system and even help protect our hearts.[67] When we laugh with others, it can improve our relationships, but even laughing alone watching a funny TV show can have benefits. It is an excellent and very enjoyable way to reduce stress that's built up in our bodies.

Crying is another important and accessible way to rid our bodies of stress, and studies have shown that it has a self-soothing effect which releases tension and enhances our mood.[68] Sometimes I find it's the only thing that will help me move on from feeling stuck in the stress surging around my body. The shower and the car are my two favourite places to have a big old cry. They feel safe and private. I find the hot water of the shower soothing once I have finished getting all the tears out. The car is great for when I know I need a cry before I get on with my day. If I have had a particularly tough morning managing everything at home and I'm exhausted from a bad night, putting on some music that will be sure to trigger a cry really helps me to release the built-up tension before I face a day working with a client. Most of us don't need a study to tell us what we already know but it is easy to forget that this is a tool at our disposal that we can reach for when necessary.

Children both cry and laugh a lot more frequently than adults do, appearing to use those tools quite naturally to soothe themselves. As adults we probably need to remind ourselves consciously that we could use a little more of both in our lives.

Animals can be an excellent source of stress reduction, and having a pet can provide both the calming sensory aspect of stroking an animal as well as companionship and a benefit to everyone in the family; a dog will also encourage you to walk outside regularly, and that can be a tonic too. While getting outside is important, it doesn't have to be grand. A weekend away in the countryside or by the sea is a wonderful thing, but spending time in any green space like a city park or our own back gardens can also have a positive effect on our mood and levels of stress. Suzy Reading calls it Nature Therapy.[69] For Suzy, after regaining some of her energy, the next important step became spending time outside every day. Living in Sydney, she could walk along the cliffs with her baby daughter and spend a little time watching the ocean. It had a powerful effect on her mood and made those trips back into the hospital to support her father much more manageable.

One friend who is also raising an autistic child combines her love of exercise with the extreme challenge of ocean swimming. It has the multiple benefits of exercise, spending time in nature and a sense of purpose she gets from both completing difficult challenges and raising money for charity.

Journaling

Journaling has been something I have returned to time and again. A year and a half after my mother died I was living in New York during 9/11 and its aftermath. It is hard to describe the palpable stress and anxiety that sat within everyone in the city at that time, even those not directly affected. I was living with a friend who was a freelance writer and she gave me a copy of *The Artist's Way* by Julia Cameron. The book is a course to discovering or rediscovering your creativity, and one of its main tools is morning pages. Cameron recommends writing three freehand, stream-of-consciousness pages each morning, dumping everything on the page to clear your head before the day begins. I found it utterly addictive. As she explains in her book, you cannot write every day and still avoid the issues that you need to deal with. Somehow, along the way, we answer our own questions and face up to our feelings, our priorities and our values. You can't hide on those pages. The key is to not reread them. Journaling is not a performative exercise. It is simply to get the words out, so we can process what is going on in our minds.

Although I no longer do morning pages first thing in the morning – impossible to do in our house – journaling as a practice is something I know I always have for when I need to work things out that are rolling around in my head. It took me a while to start journaling again after becoming a mother. For a long time I told myself I couldn't do it because I didn't have the time and space to do it as I had previously. But eventually I did start carving out little pockets of time and used it to process what was going on with Arthur's diagnosis, the renewed feelings of grief that came up about my mother and the end of my marriage. Studies have shown that writing about traumatic experiences can have a positive effect on our health.[70] I have stacks of notebooks that I don't look back at. They have served their purpose.

Stacey Leigh, whose six-year-old son Jacob is autistic, discovered journaling a little over a year ago after experiencing severe carer burnout. With the help of a psychiatrist, she began to put things into place that helped process feelings she had been ignoring for years. After Jacob's diagnosis aged two, Stacey Leigh had gone into overdrive, looking for the best ways to support him – she found him the best pre-school and then school – all while sharing her experiences online and supporting other parents going through the same process. Journaling was one of the tools recommended by her psychiatrist to help process her feelings about the diagnosis as well as some childhood trauma that she had long hidden from, in her intense pursuit to give her son the best support possible. Now she uses the technique daily. First thing in the morning she simply asks herself how she's feeling and writes for a short time about the emotions that come up. In the evenings, she journals briefly before bed, setting out any worries she has so that her mind is clearer for sleeping. Stacey Leigh says the simple act of naming her emotions on paper has changed everything for her, after years of hiding from them.

Boundaries

Self-care goes beyond the activities and skills we add to our day; it can also be about the boundaries we set up for ourselves. It can be hard to navigate this, especially in new care-giving situations, where we may have to adjust what our entire lives look like. Perhaps we had boundaries before but they all blew up when our lives took a turn. We cannot necessarily control certain boundaries when providing support for someone else. Imagine a soon-to-be parent saying, 'Well, my weekend lie-ins are just really important to me, so I'm going to keep doing that when we have kids.' Ha! But that doesn't mean we should abandon *all* boundaries. Perhaps it means saying no to a lot of other things you would have done for others in the past.

I'm not nearly as involved in either of my children's schools as I would have chosen to be if my circumstances were different. My daughter does not get driven to multiple extra-curricular activities each weekend. Her activities must be done through school or alongside a friend whose parents are happy to help. I cannot run a lot of errands with my son without it ending in disaster, nor can I pack too many social commitments in. Our weekends are slow and manageable. My garden, as much as I love it, is a bloody mess. No matter how much one of the neighbours in my street likes to cheerfully (or if I'm being less generous, passive aggressively) comment on the state of my front garden, I hold firm to the fact that I am not superwoman and my sanity is worth more than attempting to keep everyone else in our street happy.

One of my rock-solid boundaries has been to continue working. It hasn't always been easy. I have been let down by paid carers, juggled sick kids, had no access to traditional childcare settings for my son and had to work 10-hour days after getting only a couple of hours of sleep. But being in work has allowed me to explore my interests beyond my children. It allows me to pay for extra support so I'm not the only one caring for my son, which takes a lot of pressure off me. I can pay into a pension and it has also meant my children see me accept help from others – something I rarely saw in my own childhood. Even my commute to my office, a 40-minute walk through quiet back streets and a large leafy park, brings so much pleasure and sense of space to my day. A quiet commute to either day dream or listen to a book or podcast can be a wonderful opportunity to grab a moment of peace when no one, either children or work, needs anything from me. While I have no idea what the future holds for us, continuing to work will always be a top priority for me. I may just have to remain flexible about what that work looks like.

For Alice Bennett (see Chapter 1, page 28) it has meant the opposite. Alice trained as a teaching assistant, and when her daughter Raya began school, she found a job in another school, supporting disabled children. Without access to appropriate childcare for Raya, Alice felt her only option at the time was to work somewhere she would have the same term-time schedule as her daughter. After a year Alice was burned out and her mental health was suffering. It was impossible to be a present and loving caregiver at home to her two girls alongside the demands on her all day in a school. As much as she wanted to work, Alice decided it was best to quit, and she has returned to studying for now. This time Alice is not rushing and is giving herself plenty of time to figure out what is going to work best for her and her family in the future. For now, giving herself permission to study is a big step towards caring for herself.

Stacey Leigh began sharing her and her son's journey online soon after he received an autism diagnosis. She quickly attracted a lot of followers and hundreds of direct private messages, which she diligently answered. Eventually, burned out from caring at home and sharing so much with strangers, she closed her accounts and took months offline. After the break she realised that the problem had not been sharing parts of their story, but doing it with no boundaries. She has reopened a different, much smaller account where she now doesn't rush to reply to anyone she doesn't know directly, allowing it to wait until she has the time and energy. As a former social worker as well as a parent carer, she may have plenty helpful information to share, but she looks back now and can't quite believe how much time she was giving to strangers at the expense of her own health.

David Rogers, whose wife Rae has Alzheimer's (see Chapter 5, page 123) loves playing the piano. Rae tends to sleep late in the mornings, so David bought himself a keyboard with headphones and gets up early to practise for an hour without disturbing her. As the disease has progressed there is a lot that they have had to stop doing, including eating out and spending as much time with friends and grandchildren, all of which can be very distressing for Rae. Figuring out a solution that has enabled David to continue with a much-loved hobby has been essential for his wellbeing. He also plays tennis weekly and goes to the gym regularly while one of his children or a paid carer looks after Rae. These are the three things he decided would be his non-negotiables if he was to continue caring for Rae at home.

Creating time for ourselves as carers can be a tough boundary to set. While so much is possible in tiny snippets of time, we can also work towards creating more time for ourselves. Until my daughter started school, no matter what, Friday had been my day with her. It was a hugely precious time for us to enjoy activities that were either too difficult to manage with my son or were things he had no interest in. When she began school it was sad to say goodbye to that routine, but I made the decision to be proactive about ring-fencing that time for me. Before it could be swallowed up with more carer responsibilities, life admin, work admin and house-work, I set aside half the day to concentrate on writing. It would have been easy to not allow myself the time. As a single parent, a freelancer and a carer, there is a never-ending list of things to do that never go away. I had to make a decision about what was going to sustain me in the long run and decided that a tidier house and garden, a smaller washing pile and more organised admin was not going to do that. I had to do something for me.

Now that both of my children attend different schools, we have the upside of them having separate inset days (teacher training days). Each inset day, I bunk off work and spend one-to-one time with whoever is off. Agnes and I always go to the cinema or a museum, both of which Arthur struggles with. Arthur and I go trampolining or to soft play, where he can have my full attention and I'm not trying to look after the needs of them both. It is a boundary I have been able to maintain, mostly because of the flexible nature of my work. It feels like the ultimate luxury as a single parent to have one-on-one time with each child. But when you have children with very different needs from each other, it can be a boundary that's really worth holding firm to.

Creating time for ourselves, resting and prioritising our own health and wellbeing is all very well but there are times when even these, no matter how diligent we are, simply won't be enough. Humans are social creatures first and foremost, and while our caring roles may at times isolate us, our need for connection is as important as eating and breathing. We cannot get by on self-care alone, we need to be cared for. We also need to allow ourselves not just time to recuperate and re-energise, but to be our whole selves, beyond our roles as caregivers. Having a strong sense of purpose outside our immediate roles as carers can be a way of remembering who we are in the midst of an overwhelming situation. Many people find that it's actually their role as a carer that has opened them up to a purpose that they hadn't previously considered, and I'll explore this idea further in a later chapter.

Having a list of tools to turn to, as well as having regular breaks and rest, can make a huge difference to our wellbeing. But in the middle of the night, when my son is struggling, I can't just tell him that I need to take a moment for myself. There are going to be times when the needs of our parent, or partner or child are so acute that we must be fully present with them, no matter what. Times when no one else is there to take over and we must support someone else, no matter how exhausted or stressed we are. And there will be times when no matter how well rested we are, supporting another person through physical pain or extreme emotional distress will be heartbreakingly difficult. I have moments when I am on my knees, overwhelmed by my son's needs and all the while beating myself up for not handling our situation better because I had a break the day before, so I *should* be able to cope. It was only when I discovered the concept of self-compassion that I truly understood why self-care alone will *never* be enough. Eight hours of sleep a night does not mean we won't get overwhelmed or angry or emotionally burned out from providing support for another person. If we are to truly accept our situation and embrace all of its parts, we must learn to have compassion for ourselves in those moments when what is needed from us is overwhelming. For me this has been one of the hardest lessons of all.

CHAPTER 7

Self-Compassion

'When we treat others with respect and caring, the best in them usually comes out. Much the same would happen if we could treat ourselves the same way.'

Rick Hanson, psychologist and author

It is mid-morning and we are driving home from the park. I drive slowly and cautiously through back streets, forcing myself to take deep breaths, not bothering to stop the tears that keep streaming down my face. In the backseat Arthur is repeating lines from Peppa Pig to himself quietly. I could feel him getting more and more agitated at the playground. The repetitive sprinkling of sand had become larger handfuls now being thrown around. In the end a toddler got too close to him and Arthur sent her flying. Screams and apologies followed. Arthur was so distressed at this point that I had to get him away from there. I picked him up, much harder now at ten then it was when he was small, and I struggled to get us both to the car. We were near a busy road and if I put him down I knew he would run blind into it. He was thrashing and trying to get away from me but I knew now, having been through this so many times, that the car would calm him and make him feel safe. I stayed focused, ignoring the looks from strangers.

As soon as the seat-belt is in place, his body starts to relax and his breathing begins to slow. Within minutes he's calmed and is asking for a snack and some water. I fumble around in my bag for the emergency snacks that are always there. Crunchy foods that are both satisfying and calming to his nervous system. My head aches where his flailing limbs hit me. I look at him in the rear-view mirror as I drive. He looks at me and says, 'Hello Mummy' with a small smile. I put my sunglasses on so he doesn't notice the tears falling uncontrollably down my face. I don't want him to think it's his fault that I'm upset. I know he had no control over his actions a few moments ago. His ability to recover from a meltdown always astonishes me. While I have learned to stay focused and calm for him when he's struggling, as soon as the danger has passed I want to fall to pieces. No matter what I have done that day to care for myself, the breaks I have had, the decent night's sleep I managed, while it all helps, in these moments it disappears. I am reminded that sometimes it's just hard. It's hard to watch him struggle. It's getting harder to carry him to safety. And fear rears up about how I will handle a situation like this in the future, when he's taller and bigger than me.

Self-criticism

I have never felt as powerless as when my son is in the throes of a meltdown. I'm often able to de-escalate it before it gets that far, but sometimes it is beyond my control. Seeing someone you love in such emotional turmoil feels impossible some days. And yet I know that if I stay calm for him, I can help him through it faster than if I get worked up. Rationally it makes complete sense. Practically, it can feel like a herculean effort. There have been days when we are both left sobbing and hugging on the floor, my internal monologue a barrage of criticism for all the things I didn't do right in the moment. I *should* have stayed calm. I *shouldn't* have raised my voice. I *shouldn't* have left that plate sitting on the table. And right back it goes to all the possible things I had done wrong that day that meant he hasn't coped.

I'm certainly not alone in struggling with difficult feelings as a carer. Some people may feel resentful that other family members aren't doing their share. Others may feel too much has been asked of them and may be angry that they have given up work, or time with other family and friends. Jealousy of other people's freedom and time for themselves, helplessness that they are witnessing pain that they can't fix, loneliness because the person they support can't communicate the way they used to. There can be so many conflicting and difficult emotions going on, even in situations where a person has chosen to be the main carer, and it can all lead to a lot of self-criticism.

Self-criticism is not at all unusual. We all have an inner critic. For most of us it is a voice that is easy to recall in our minds. We barely have to think back and we remember times when our loud inner critic decided it must be heard. Work, relationships, body image, physical abilities, intelligence or parenting, we all have a hard and nasty voice that pipes up when we feel we could do better, be better, behave better. We have another voice, though. One that is sometimes quieter and less familiar to us. But it can be encouraged and cultivated. Despite what our instincts may tell us, it can also be far more motivating than our inner critic. It is our compassionate voice.

What is self-compassion?

Dr Kristin Neff, an Associate Professor of Human Development and Culture at the University of Texas at Austin, came across the Buddhist concept of self-compassion during her post-doctoral work on self-esteem. The research she had done into self-esteem showed that it had some downsides. It was often dependent on the need to be above average and it could lead to social comparison, prejudice and narcissism. Self-compassion, on the other hand, appeared to boost not self-esteem but intrinsic self-worth. Dr Neff writes that self-esteem relies on evaluating ourselves in comparison to others, but self-compassion is not based on evaluation and judgment: you don't have to feel better than others to feel good about yourself. When she found that were no academic studies on the effects of self-compassion, she began to research it herself. She published her first paper in 2003 and there are now thousands of published studies on the subject. It became clear to Dr Neff as she deepened her research that there is a strong link between self-compassion and wellbeing.[71] People who are high in self-compassion are less depressed, less stressed and less anxious. It is associated with less self-criticism,[72] less rumination on negative thoughts[73] and a better ability to bounce back after negative moods.[74] High levels of self-compassion have also been found to be associated with increased happiness, optimism, life satisfaction and motivation.[75] But what exactly is self-compassion?

There are three main elements that Dr Neff defined in her initial research. The first is mindfulness, or the ability to be aware of our moment-to-moment experience. This is important because we must be aware of our suffering in order to turn towards it with kindness. This can take the form of simply acknowledging to ourselves how we feel. The second element is common humanity. This is the very important acknowledgement that suffering, difficult feelings and things going wrong are things that we all experience as humans. It is about remembering that we are not alone in our pain but rather that it connects us with others. It is all too easy to feel isolated when we are suffering, but nothing is more universal or more human. The third element is self-kindness. While it may feel very natural to criticise ourselves for mistakes and failures, instead we can choose to treat ourselves as we would a good friend. With warmth and kindness, offering support and care instead of harsh criticism.

But it wasn't just the research that got me really interested in Dr Neff's work, rather it was the personal circumstances in which she found herself that had me stop and pay more attention. In 2007 her son Rowan was diagnosed with autism and it was her self-compassion practice that got her through. Initially, it helped her process all her difficult feelings. She allowed herself to feel without judgment. The fear and sadness coupled with the deep sense of shame that she felt at having such feelings around the most important person in the world to her. As she met each of her feelings with compassion, she very quickly found that with this practice, she had the resources to be the unconditionally loving parent she wanted to be for Rowan. With self-compassion she could weather the storms of public meltdowns and stay loving and present with Rowan, despite nasty looks from strangers. She could face criticism for her parenting from people who didn't understand and she could bounce back from mistakes more quickly, better able to refocus her support on her son who needed her. It gave her the ability to be the caregiver she wanted to be.

When I read about her experiences I knew that I had to give self-compassion a proper go – to see if it would alleviate some of the difficulties around caring and the deep desire I had to be more present with my son when he was having a really hard time.

Do I deserve compassion?

The first roadblock I came to when I began to explore the idea of self-compassion was, did I even deserve it? When my son is struggling, he's the one who needs compassion, not me. And would losing my self-criticism after a meltdown mean I would be less likely to look for better preventative measures to help Arthur? Dr Chris Germer, co-author with Dr Neff of *The Mindful Self-Compassion Program*, says there are a lot of myths around about self-compassion that we need to address before we can get in the habit of using it. He says that there is a deep suspicion of self-compassion in Western culture, that to be kind to ourselves is too self-focused and selfish. We fear that being kind to ourselves will lead to self-pity, or that it will soften us when we need to remain strong. The most common misconception, he says, is that people worry that they won't be motivated to do better if they are always kind to themselves when they fail or make mistakes.[76] I was certainly not alone in my fears about being kinder to myself.

Dr Neff developed a self-compassion scale, which leads you through a series of questions designed to reveal the level of your self-compassion. It gives you a final ranking which puts you at either low, medium or high levels of self-compassion. Multiple studies have shown that rather than leading to complacency, self-compassion can enhance motivation. It's been found that people high in self-compassion hold themselves to high standards[77] and engage in less self-sabotaging behaviours such as procrastination.[78] They also suffer less from imposter syndrome[79] and have less fear about failing.[80] When people high in self-compassion do fail, they are more likely to try again.[81] One interesting study found that people were more likely to apologise for a behaviour they regretted and felt bad about, if they were helped to be more self-compassionate.[82] Far from letting ourselves off the hook by going 'easy' on ourselves, self-compassion can enhance our resilience and grit in the face of failure[83] without excusing bad behaviour.

As for whether offering ourselves compassion makes us more selfish, the opposite appears to be true. Self-compassionate people tend to be more caring and supportive in their relationships. A person who is able to give themselves compassion has more resources available to them to offer support to their partners.[84] They are also better able to have perspective on a problem and spend less time in rumination, which makes them *less* rather than more self-absorbed.

More specifically, a study of people caring for a loved one with dementia showed that self-compassion was associated with less caregiver burnout.[85] Another study of parents of autistic children found that those with high levels of self-compassion were less stressed and less depressed than those with lower levels of self-compassion. It also found that self-compassion was a stronger predictor for how well a parent adjusted to the diagnosis than the severity of the child's disability. This suggests that how a person relates to themselves is more important than the severity of the challenges they face as a carer.[86]

An informal self-compassion practice

The next time my son was having a really hard time, I promised myself I would give it a try. I didn't have to wait long before we had a 2am start one morning. Exhausted, stressed about the amount of work I had ahead of me that day, fed up and resentful of feeling so tired, I was much grumpier and speaking more curtly with Arthur than I usually would. My usual self-criticism kicked in, telling me I was being a terrible mother, that he can't help his sleeplessness, that it's not his fault I have to work, that I should know better than to be snappy with him. But remembering my promise to try something different, I stopped. I tried what Dr Germer describes as a self-compassion break, an informal practice recommended for when you are struggling.

The first step is noticing the feelings. I started silently naming my feelings to myself, as Arthur sat beside me eating a very early breakfast. I'm so tired. I'm worried I won't get my work done. I'm scared that my health will suffer from lack of sleep. I worry about getting ill because how will I look after Arthur then? I worry that Arthur will think my bad mood is his fault. It was interesting just naming all those feelings. One by one they popped up in my mind, one leading to another. Wow, I thought to myself, I'm really worried about a lot of things.

The second step is to remember our common humanity, that I was not alone in feeling like this. I imagined it was a friend telling me these worries. They wouldn't seem insignificant, they would be understandable. Lots of people would find a 2am start hard.

The third and final step is to offer yourself kindness. This is hard, I found myself saying in my head. This is hard for Arthur *and* for me. I'm not a bad mother for finding this hard. It's ok to find this hard. You're doing your best. As I sat with those thoughts for a few minutes, I snuggled in to Arthur. The resentment felt a bit less. The guilt at having ugly feelings felt a bit less too. I was still really tired but I felt less anxious about my tiredness. Arthur smiled at me and said 'Hello Mummy! Morning!' in his usual very loud and chirpy voice that seemed even louder and chirpier at this time of the night. I smiled and sighed: 'I suppose it is morning,' I said.

As my attempts at offering myself compassion increased, I noticed something interesting. I didn't get angry, upset or annoyed less often but I did seem to come out of stewing in these feelings much faster. I still felt guilty when I didn't respond to Arthur in the way I thought he deserved, but somehow the guilt didn't always morph into shame as it had so often before. I felt bad that I didn't respond the way I wanted, but I didn't tell myself I was a terrible mother for doing so. I bounced back more quickly and was more ready to apologise if I felt I had been less patient with him than I should have been. And when I responded to my difficult feelings with kindness I felt a sense of ease that was familiar. The kind of ease that comes from a good friend listening to my worries. Except I could be alone in my house with Arthur at 4am and be offering it to myself instead of waiting hours till I saw a familiar face. It didn't stop the pain of witnessing Arthur struggle, or stop feelings of exhaustion, but it did seem to bring comfort where I struggled to find comfort before. It finally occurred to me that I had spent years not considering I was allowed to have my own feelings while I supported someone else through theirs.

As my mother had got increasingly unwell in my early teens, I learned to hide my emotions from her. My feelings made her worse, that was clear to me. She was so wrapped up in her own depression that she had no space for any feelings I might have. If I let those feelings out, hers overflowed too. There were times when my own emotions led hers to become so unmanageable that she ended up in hospital. Looking back, as an adult, I can see what an impossible and unsustainable situation we were in. It wasn't my mother's fault that she was too unwell to support me, and I was very young to be supporting her through depression when I had no one else looking after me on a day-to-day basis. This is a situation so many young carers face. They must be the support for others when they are in desperate need themselves. The more I read about self-compassion, the more I realised I that although as a practice it was new to me, as a concept and a way of looking after myself I had used it before. I just didn't have the words to describe it back then.

When things get really difficult

When I was 14, things at home became extremely difficult. My mum was struggling and was in and out of a psychiatric unit a number of times that year. It was just my middle brother Pip and me living at home with her, with a paid carer coming in to support Mum a few hours a couple of times a week. Maureen was an ex-mental-health nurse and came in to help out around the house and be someone for my mum to lean on. She was a wonderfully warm and no-nonsense woman who left us casseroles in the fridge to heat up and remind us we were not alone.

I was waiting at the train station one day after a late finish at school. I was angry at the fact Mum had yet again forgotten to collect me after promising she would be here. No matter how many times I was let down, when she promised me she would be somewhere, I couldn't help but hope she would. I used the phone box to call the house but there was no answer. I tried again and again and eventually Maureen answered. She told me that she would come and get me herself but that I should start walking anyway and she would meet me halfway. I hung up angrier than I had been before. The walk was a few miles and Maureen wouldn't tell me why Mum wasn't coming. About 20 minutes into my walk home, she pulled up in my mother's car and let me in. She told me, in her matter-of-fact manner, that she had arrived that afternoon to find my mother had attempted suicide, and when I had called the ambulance was still there. She had made me walk to delay me. She didn't want me to see her in the state she was in.

For the rest of that year, when I woke up each morning and when I got home from school each day, I crept into my mother's room, where she was often still in bed, and checked to see if she was breathing. I became so accustomed to doing it, it barely registered any more. There were days when I arrived home and something would look different. The French doors to the garden would be wide open, or the car would be gone. I would begin to call out for her, my heart beating faster, trying not to panic. When I would find her in bed, snoring, or wandering around the garden drunk, I would release the breath I had been holding. Every day I expected to find her dead. Each day that I found her alive I felt an enormous sense of relief. But it wouldn't last long. It would slowly build up until I was again walking around the house after school, not daring to breathe. I had a deep sense that this couldn't go on, but, at the same time, I couldn't see how it would end either.

Over the Christmas break, my dad took us to visit family outside of Sydney where, without realising I was even looking for one, a solution presented itself to me. We spent some time with distant cousins we hadn't seen in a while, one of whom had been away to boarding school. It was a different kind of school to the one my brother had gone to while we had lived on the farm. You went for a whole term, only getting one weekend off to go home, rather than going home every Friday night. I hadn't known those kinds of schools existed in Australia. Back at home with Mum in Melbourne, with things returning to the usual difficult routine, it occurred to me that maybe it didn't have to be this way. My brother's weekly school situation hadn't appealed to me particularly. But the idea of really going away, properly away, suddenly felt like it might be a very good idea. When Dad came to collect me for dinner one evening, I asked him what he thought. He looked hugely relieved and said yes right away. I realised much later that I had presented him with something he could actually do to help, in a situation where no one really knew what to do to

help us. Living with my dad had never been an option – he travelled far too much and spent most of his time abroad. But if I
was willing to go away to school, he was willing to pay. I knew
even back then of the huge privilege I had, that my dad could
afford to send me away like that. But I also knew the cost was
going to be far more than just financial.

My mother was furious. The day she found out she looked me
in the eyes and told me it would be my fault if she died. That I
had abandoned her. I sobbed and begged for her to understand
how things were for me, and it only made things worse. She
called me selfish and ungrateful and every ugly word I could have
imagined. It was less than three weeks to the start of term and
the school had told my dad they had a place for me if I wanted
it. But Mum told me I should pack my bags and leave that day. In
a panic about what I had done I called my aunt Janine, and not
long after, both of my mum's sisters arrived, along with my eldest
cousin. After first attempting to calm my mother down, Janine
came to see me in my room. I thought she was going to ask me to
change my mind. I expected them to be so worried about my
mum that they would do anything to support her. Instead, she
calmly looked at me, with her hands on each of my arms and
said: 'I know this must be hard but you're doing the right thing.'

It was the first time I became conscious of the weight I had
been carrying on my shoulders. The countless times I had been
there for my mum, holding her hand when there had been no one
there to hold mine. My mother had been ship-wrecked, clinging
on to me like a life raft and, without meaning to, she was dragging me under. Somehow, instinct had told me that I was drown-
ing and that it was time I saved myself. When my dad and my
aunts stepped in to defend me, it was like I could see that clearly
for the first time. I could see that no matter what I did, I was not
going to be able save my mother. Whether she lived or died,

whether she recovered or not, it wasn't within my control. No amount of sitting by her bedside or checking she was still breathing would change things for her. But I could save myself.

Over the following week my mother gradually calmed down. She was still angry at me and we barely spoke. When my new uniform arrived and my bags were all packed, I left not knowing whether what I was about to do would be the last straw for her. In those first few weeks as I settled in to school, made new friends and learned my way around, I waited every day for a phone call that would tell me she was dead. Eventually when the phone call didn't come, I began to relax a little. It was the first time I was completely conscious of how much I had been doing for myself for the previous couple of years. At school I had three hot meals cooked for me a day and someone checking I attended those meals. I was forced to participate in sport and after-school activities, something I hadn't done in years. Someone made sure I went to class and I was surrounded by friends, all day every day. The full realisation of how isolated I had become looking after Mum hit me. While many friends moaned about being at boarding school, I thrived. It had been so long since I had felt that well cared for.

When I arrived home after my first term, my mother was in a great mood. We sat at our kitchen counter and talked for hours over a meal she had cooked for me especially. I told her all of the details about my new life that I hadn't gone into over the telephone. My friends, the classes, the bizarre rituals of boarding school. At the end of the night as I went off to bed, she hugged me and told me I had done the right thing. She told me she hadn't seen me like this in such a long time, so happy, so my old self, that she had almost forgotten what I was like. She told me she was proud of me for leaving. While I was so happy to hear those words, I also knew to take everything she now told me with a pinch of salt. The next drunken rant she had at me, she went right back to blaming her problems on me for leaving her, and the argument went on for many years. She would pick fights with me the night before I returned to school each term, like clockwork. But I knew that when she was in her right mind, when she was sober and thoughtful, she was glad that I had chosen to put myself first.

Though I continued to wait for that phone call, and remained jumpy whenever a teacher requested a private conversation, I felt incredibly supported at school. I'm not sure how much of the details of my home life my house mistress knew, but she was like a rock during those years. I continued supporting mum from a distance, over the phone, but it was now within my control when I spoke to her. I still spent all my holidays with her, offering bedside support as I had done before. My brother Pip had hated the idea of boarding school and he had stayed at home. But he never seemed resentful for me leaving when I did. But not everyone was understanding about what I had chosen to do; during my first holiday back at home an old school friend of mine asked after Mum and when I replied that she wasn't doing very well, she looked at me and said, 'well, what do you expect. You left her.' Although I felt a deep sense of shame in that moment, I felt something else as well. Even after one term I knew I had done the right thing. I had been headed for burnout at home. Had I stayed, I'm not sure if I could have survived high school with my mental health intact and good enough grades to get into university. Leaving had saved me, and even as early as that first term I knew it had.

I look back now on the decision I made for myself just before I turned 15 and I can see that it was my first deliberate act of self-compassion. Every decision I have made for myself since that day has not been as difficult as the one when I chose to put my own needs before my mother's. I realise now that without being able to offer myself kindness at the time, I would never have been able to take a step back from being my mother's main support. Without self-compassion, I wouldn't have believed I deserved a chance to finish high school without the constant responsibility of looking after my mother, as well as myself, while she went through a period of severe mental illness.

Soft and fierce

Although the practice of *soft* self-compassion was new to me as a parent, offering myself kindness when I failed, I realised I had been practising fierce self-compassion for many years already. Dr Neff describes compassion as comprising a yin and a yang. The soft yin of self-compassion is in comforting, soothing and validating ourselves. The fierce yang of self-compassion is in protecting, providing and motivating. It is what we need to set strong boundaries and stand up for ourselves and others we care for. We need both of these aspects of self-compassion.

Carers become well used to being called on to use fierce self-compassion when they stand up for themselves and their loved ones in social care assessments, medical appointments and elsewhere in the community; when they say 'enough is enough' and demand more support, going to court if necessary to get it. Fierce self-compassion is insisting on some much-needed respite, even when it's uncomfortable for the person you support. It's in insisting that your needs are as important as your partner's, parent's or child's. They may not be as acute but they are equal.

A simple breathing exercise

While soft self-compassion may not come very easily to me, I have continued to practise it. When we are struggling through a hard day, when all else is failing, I now fall back on the technique of equanimity breathing that Dr Neff describes using during her own son's meltdowns. Sometimes, in a hard moment supporting someone else, all you can do is breathe. I take in a deep breath, offering myself compassion and kind words. As I breathe out, I send kindness and compassion towards my son. And back and forth it goes, one in-breath for me and one out for him, until my mind is quieter and my body is calmer.

Feelings of compassion aren't necessarily easy to summon up if we aren't used to being compassionate towards ourselves. Dr Neff recommends bringing the face of a dear friend to mind, someone who you have warm feelings for and an easy relationship with. Ask yourself, how would you treat that friend if they were going through what you are going through?

It's uncomfortable at first. Why should I breathe in for myself, I think, when my son is struggling so much? Because this is hard for me too, I remind myself, as I continue to breathe in and out. Compassion is not finite. Taking a breath in for me doesn't take anything away from Arthur. Self-compassion, as many studies have shown, breeds compassion for others. The more I can give to myself, the more I have to give Arthur. It's omnidirectional.

Dr Neff recommends that for both unpaid and paid carers (such as nurses, doctors and paramedics), it's a good idea to have a few informal practices to use when things are extremely challenging and you can't take a break. She calls these 'on the job' practices.

Supportive touch technique

As well as the self-compassion break and the breathing technique above, another technique is supportive touch. This is where we use our own touch to activate the parasympathetic nervous system to help calm us down when we are stressed. It works in exactly the same way as when someone else gives us soothing touch, such as a hug. Amazingly, our bodies don't know the difference. It's good to know that in really difficult moments, this is something we can do for ourselves. Some people find this feels really strange and awkward, but with practice it can begin to feel as natural as touching someone else when they are having a hard time, like putting a hand on their shoulder.

Begin by taking a few deep breaths and then experiment with putting your hand on different parts of your body, to see which feels more comfortable to you. Some people find putting their hand over their heart works well for them. Others prefer a hand on their cheek, cupping one hand over the other in your lap, or crossing your arms and giving yourself a gentle squeeze. There are many other techniques and practices that can be found for free on Dr Neff's website and in both her and Dr Germer's books (see the resources section on page 251 for more information).

The paradox of self-compassion

When I spoke to Dr Germer about the self-compassion break and how I often find it works well, he smiled warmly and then reminded me the point was not that it should 'work'. He explained that if we get caught up in the idea that self-compassion 'fixes' a situation for us, we are going to end up being frustrated and disillusioned. The central paradox of self-compassion is that if we practise it in order to solve a problem, it won't work because it is not a problem-solving technique. But if we offer ourselves compassion because we are human and we are suffering, then it will, in turn, ease our suffering. It is a tricky concept to get my head around but he used a great analogy to help me understand. He told me to imagine your child is sick with a five-day flu. Lots of kids in the neighbourhood have had it, you know it's not serious and your child will be fine after five days. You comfort your child, you cuddle them and bring them food and drink that might make them feel a bit more comfortable; you might read to them and offer lots of reassuring words. You do this because your child is suffering with the flu. You don't do this because you think it will make the flu instantly go away. You already know, based on all the other kids that have had it, that it will still take five days, whether you are kind to your child or not. You are kind and loving towards your child because they deserve kindness when they are unwell. Dr Germer says offering kindness to ourselves works in exactly the same way. Suffering is unavoidable as a human. We might pretend that this isn't true but to be human means things will go wrong, we will experience pain and failure and so will those we love. This, Dr Germer says, is reason enough to offer ourselves kindness.

Acceptance of difficulties

Accepting that life can be uncomfortable, painful and difficult sometimes, seems to be a key aspect to bringing some ease to a hard situation. At times, when I am having a hard day, not necessarily to do with my son having a very hard time but when everything is compounded by having to argue for my son's needs and access rights in meetings, feeling like I'm beating my head against a brick wall of austerity, I try to stop everything momentarily. As I take a moment to breathe, I ask myself: what is it that

I want from my life? Do I just want an easy life? When I phrase it like that, I remember that I did not sign up for an easy life. I made the choice to have an adventurous life. If I had wanted an easy life I would have stayed in the city I was born, I would have had a dependable and safe job and I would not have had children. Even as those little lines showed up on the pregnancy test almost 11 years ago, I knew in that moment the potential pain I was opening myself up to. Every parent must accept that, just as every human who loves another human must accept that with love there is the possibility of loss and pain. This is not something I always want to accept. Sometimes it just feels so unfair that we must fight for basic services, or that my son struggles with things many find so straightforward.

Not wanting to accept things as they are is often referred to as resistance. Where we resist, we increase our suffering. Dr Neff describes resistance as the belief that our moment-to-moment experience should be other than it is.[87] But acceptance of our situations is not the same as passively accepting a government that is damaging the lives of disabled people and those who support them, or assuming that I won't find more creative solutions to some of my son's challenges. Acceptance means not layering further suffering on top of painful aspects that are a natural fact of life. This is where the practice of mindfulness seems to be particularly helpful. When we can identify how we feel, without judging ourselves, we can begin to let those feelings go. Research has shown that when we try to suppress feelings and thoughts that we don't like or find challenging, they just get stronger.[88] But when we bring mindfulness to our situation we can begin to accept those feelings, and when we add compassion, that can bring some ease. As Dr Neff writes: 'Mindfulness asks, "What am I *experiencing* right now?", self-compassion asks, "What do I *need* right now?"'[89]

What is the kindest thing I can do for myself right now?

'What is the kindest thing I can do for myself right now?' is a question I am getting in the habit of asking myself during difficult times. Sometimes that answer is a very early night, reaching out to a friend, going for a run or skipping a run and going back to bed. It's not always what is easiest or what I want, but what is *kindest*. When I treat myself with kindness, I find the energy to advocate better for Arthur, and I even find more patience on the hard days too. I can look back at the decision I made to go away to school when I was 14 and I can now see that what I did was an act of kindness to myself. How I knew to do that for myself I still don't know. Just as arguing for respite hours through social care to help me through the long summer holidays, many carers will at some point be faced with needing to put their own needs first and demanding some support.

How much support and when is so individual that there can be no right and wrong. For some it may be making the difficult decision to stop being the main caregiver and find a suitable care home to better meet the around-the-clock-care needs of a parent or partner. It may mean a massive increase in the number of paid carers coming into your home to support your loved one, whether they're happy about it or not. Sometimes the most compassionate thing a carer can do is take a step back and ask for more support. When approached from a place of self-compassion, we may be able to fight for what we need before we become so burned out we are not able to care for the person we are supporting.

As I write, it has been around 18 months since I started improving my self-compassion skills. Some days it feels like I have a long way to go. But as I came to write this chapter, I was curious as to the progress I had made. I retook the self-compassion test (available for free online)[90] and afterwards I pulled out the previous test I had taken 18 months earlier, a paper version I had folded and put into a notebook. I had gone from scoring medium to high in self-compassion in that period of time. I scanned over the answers I had given and could see areas where there was a marked improvement, particularly around self-criticism and how long it took me to bounce back from difficult moments. In that time I haven't done anything particularly drastic. I have mostly been trying to run through the three steps of a self-compassion break when I am really struggling: notice the feelings, find common humanity, and offer myself kindness.

It is sometimes harder than it sounds. But this simple tool has made a huge difference to how I recover from hard moments. It has meant hard moments don't turn into hard days, and hard days don't turn into hard weeks. They simply remain hard, painful moments.

CHAPTER 8

Community

'*There is nothing like puking with somebody to make you into old friends.*'[91]

Sylvia Plath

I was at my friend Marisa's house when my mother called. Marisa lived in a large unconverted warehouse near our university, with plenty of space for extras when things were too intense at home and I needed a break. I could tell Mum was bad the moment I heard her voice. I asked Marisa if she minded if we went via my house on the way to our Wednesday night dance class. Marisa knew my mum well. The downside of the cool warehouse with plenty of space was that it was absolutely freezing. During the winter that year we had decamped to my mum's plenty of times to take advantage of the central heating and the generous fridge. Marisa would share cigarettes and drink black coffee with my mum at our kitchen counter. Being the daughter of a psychiatrist and a GP, she was not afraid of my mum's honest conversations, and in fact rather enjoyed them. As we drove towards my house, I had a feeling of dread that I hadn't felt for a while. I'm not exactly sure if my mother had improved over the previous couple of years or if I had just become so accustomed to the cycles of depression and drinking that they had ceased to disturb me as much. Now an adult and in possession of a car and friends who had their own places, I could always get away when I needed to. My relationship with my mum had improved significantly because of this. But something about her tone on the phone made me feel uneasy. Memories of coming home from school and expecting to find her unconscious loomed in my mind.

When we arrived at the house, Mum was sitting at the top of the stairs, exactly opposite the front door. She was sobbing and slurring her words and fiddling with something in her lap. I told Marisa to go make some coffee and find the phone. I went up the stairs to her and sat down. She held the end of her dog Mimi's lead in her hand. It was the old-fashioned kind of lead, with a chain that pulled tight when you tugged on it. I gently loosened the chain that was looped around her neck and slipped it off over her head. She looked at me, crying and said, 'I need to go to the clinic.' I knew what she meant. She needed to be watched that night and she didn't want the responsibility on my shoulders. I told her I would sort it out and brought her down the stairs. We found her psychiatrist's number and I called her. She had received this call many times and she said she'd check for a bed and get right back to me. A few minutes later she called and said there would be no bed at the private clinic my mum usually stayed in till tomorrow but that she had found a space in the public ward. If it was urgent, she said, she urged me to take Mum in. I asked Mum what she wanted to do. She was shaking at the thought but she agreed she would go. Marisa stayed with her while I packed a bag for her.

When we arrived at the inner-city hospital I was in for a shock. My mum's foresight to get private health insurance many years before she became ill meant that despite all that I had witnessed and helped her through, I had still been largely sheltered. In a private clinic I was well aware of the variety and extreme distress experienced by many people, including girls my own age, but I hadn't been confronted with involuntary sections and closed wards. Although my mum was choosing to walk in that day, not everyone there was. The place felt Victorian, echoing with tiles and hard surfaces. I could hear shouts from closed rooms and through internal windows could see vacant men and women staring at a TV or the wall. Handing her over to the staff there, who didn't know her, when she was in the state she was in, was one of the most dreadful things I have ever done. She looked terrified. I tried to reassure her, it's just one night, I said. You'll be transferred tomorrow. She nodded and seemed more like a small child than my mother. But she knew she could not be at home that night. She knew this was her best option. The staff reassured me and ushered us out. Marisa and I went back to the car downstairs and just sat silent in it for a while. 'I don't think I can go dancing,' I told her. We drove back to the warehouse, opened a bottle of red wine and sat huddled around her old-fashioned oven that was the best source of heat in the place. We ate nachos and talked for hours. I don't even think we talked about what had happened that afternoon.

Before Marisa and I had met at university, I had plenty of friends, some of whom I'm still very close to today. But I had largely hidden my home life from everyone when I was younger. They may have known what was going on but I don't remember feeling as though I could confide in anyone. This is a particularly big problem for young carers, 89% of whom report feeling lonely and isolated.[92] I had my brothers, and it meant a lot to me just knowing they were there, but we didn't tend to talk often about our experiences with Mum. When we met in a photography class at the beginning of our first year, Marisa and I became close friends so quickly it was almost like a love affair. It wasn't long before we both discovered each of our families had their own traumas of different kinds, and perhaps that's why it was so easy to be friends. It was a relief when she dealt with my mother's ups and downs with pragmatism and empathy. She was not afraid of my mother's long and very revealing conversations over wine and cigarettes. Equally, she didn't put up with any of my mum's bullshit either, and quickly jumped to my defence if she thought my mother was being unfair or placing too high a burden on me. Perhaps it was easier living with my mum during my university years because of my age and my ability to escape when I needed to. Or perhaps it was because I had Marisa that made all the difference.

We are not meant to do this alone

Humans have evolved to live in small groups. It may feel as though the way we live now in the modern world is normal, but it's not how it has been for most of human history. Isolated in houses occupied only by immediate nuclear families, commuting long distances to work, working long hours outside of the home: these are all modern aspects of life which as humans we are not necessarily designed for. We may live in a time that is obsessed with individualism, equating it with pride, freedom and auton-omy, but we are an interdependent species. We are not built to do this alone. And yet many of us do. It is all very well to learn about how ableism has coloured our views of disability, to get enough sleep, learn about acceptance and self-compassion, but we cannot get away from the fact that we absolutely cannot do this alone. Nor are we meant to.

Finding connections as a new carer is not always easy and there can be so many barriers to finding the right support. Natalie Lee, whose daughter is visually impaired and will one day lose her sight due to a rare genetic condition, told me part of the issue has been that her daughter isn't interested. Natalie told me her daughter is not yet comfortable with her identity as a visually impaired person and has felt quite strongly that she doesn't want to spend time with other kids in her position. This can be common for many families when one family member becomes ill or disabled and is not ready to accept it or be open about it. Someone facing a life-changing diagnosis may take a long time to process it and may go through a prolonged period of grief while they let go of and even rebuild their identity. Natalie, understandably, wants to give her daughter plenty of space to decide when she's ready to be involved with other kids with a similar disability. This has meant that Nathalie and her husband haven't really connected with other parents in a similar position. Instead, they found a counsellor, someone with whom they could discuss their worries and fears.

Shared life experience

Understanding and the absence of judgment really seem to be the main benefits to seeking out a community which specifically includes other carers in a similar position. I had plenty of friends when Arthur was diagnosed, but what we were going through was so different and alien to what they were going through that it became difficult to talk about, without feeling I had to explain every little thing at length. Or caveat with reassurances of 'but I'm ok, really I'm ok,' because the looks of horror or pity or sadness on their faces were just too much to deal with on top of my own emotions. Other parent carers have told me how friends have withdrawn, not knowing what to say, or feeling like they can't ever complain about their own issues at home because they seem trivial in comparison. I often left social gatherings feeling more isolated and more alone in my problems, because anything

I had to contribute looked nothing like what anyone else was experiencing.

Part of the reason these kinds of interactions leave us feeling bad is how inauthentic they can feel. If we are brave enough to bare our souls about what is actually happening at home, the blank stares can send us right back into our box, reminding us that we are as alone as we thought we were. So we remain silent. But when we find others going through the same, the opposite can happen.

Around the time Arthur turned four I discovered our local autism parenting support group was having a Christmas party hosted by one of its members. I plucked up the courage to go alone, and walked the 15 minutes to a large home on the other side of my neighbourhood. I was welcomed in, handed a drink and instantly drawn into conversations. I left hours later, feeling like I had found my people in a way I hadn't felt in a very long time. We all howled with laughter over some of the wonderful and ridiculous things that happen in our homes, the conversations we never expected we would have and the things we never imagined we would be proud of. For the next few years a group of us would try to meet once a month for drinks. Sometimes we would swap numbers of lawyers and independent speech therapists, give tribunal advice to each other and commiserate over yet another local authority failing, or just listen to each other rant. Many other times we talked about the rest of our lives, happy in the knowledge that no background explanation was needed. As our kids get older and our lives more complicated, it's getting more challenging to meet up regularly and the WhatsApp group has to make up for when we can't all get together.

As a middle-class, English-speaking woman in a large city, finding support through groups has been relatively straightforward. Parenting support groups of all kinds tend to be a lot easier to find and tap into then other kinds of support groups.

Syreeta, whose husband Rob has a brain injury (see Chapter 4, page 100) found it impossible to find an in-person group that she had anything in common with. Every attendee was at least 30 years older than her and it was hard to find common ground. When I spoke to one of my son's therapists about how important our local support group had been, she mentioned that she had many clients who were not born in the UK who struggled to access these groups because of language or cultural differences. It's certainly not as easy as looking up what's available and making the time to attend. Support groups also mean leaving the house, which can be so difficult for many. Even though I found many people in my situation locally, my ability to attend meet-ups over white wine and crisps in the pub went dramatically downhill after becoming a single parent.

Finding community online

The rise of social media has been incredibly powerful for the disabled community. Where once you may have known no one in your own town sharing the same impairment and challenges that you do, now you can be connected with a community all over the world, regardless of location. Many of the physical barriers that prevent disabled people being able to fully participate disappear online. No need to worry about wheelchair access, parking, having to use public transport that isn't fit for purpose. No need to worry about burning yourself out, using what precious energy you have to get out of the house. No need to communicate face to face in real time, which can be problematic for many. And what has been good for disabled people has also been good for those caring for parent, partner or friend.

Whether you have a child with a rare genetic disorder or a parent or partner with Huntington's or Parkinson's, social media helps us find each other in a way that is possible like never before. If you are physically isolated because of the location you live in, or your inability to get out and about because of your caring responsibilities, the internet has opened up our worlds.

Emma Gardner, whose daughter Dotty has the rare chromosome deletion STXBP1 (see Chapter 3, page 85), did a search on Instagram by popping a hashtag in front of it. She was surprised to find lots of parents all around the world posting about life with their children who have the same condition. Even better than that, by chance she realised someone who was posting had a daughter just a little older than Dotty living a few minutes away. They started to meet up in person and were able to share lots of information. Dotty now even attends the same school. Quite incredible for a genetic condition that has a prevalence of only around 1 in 90,000.

Similarly, carers of all kinds can search and find others on social media with the same impairments or conditions as the person they support. As I suggested in Chapter 4, this is a great way to understand how to support someone better, especially if they aren't able to (or no longer able to) communicate their needs. So much of my own learning about autism and how I might better understand my son has been through the Twitter hashtag ActuallyAutistic. The hashtag is a great way to connect with and learn from people who might be able to shed more light on my son's lived experience than a teacher or medical professional can.

Many of the carers I have spoken to use closed, private Facebook groups to share information, get support and have a safe rant away from the public eye. The quality of these groups can vary, as can people's experience of them. While they can provide incredible support, they can have the downside – that all social media has – of having very strong opinions that if you don't agree with can get you kicked out or piled on by other users.

Being part of a community is easier for carers of some conditions than others. Autism, Down's syndrome and cerebral palsy have strong, if occasionally divided, communities for parent carers. Many of the carers I have spoken to in their twenties and thirties, supporting either a parent or a partner, have found online communities particularly helpful. There they can find people their own age with similar struggles as themselves. At a time in their life when most of their friends are travelling, focusing on their careers, getting married and starting families, carers in this age group can feel a great sense of loss that only other carers their own age will fully understand.

But not all disabled people have a named condition, and this can make it harder for a carer to find where they belong. Laura Godfrey, whose son Oscar is now eight, has never received an overall diagnosis. He has, like many children, what's known as a SWAN, a syndrome without a name. Over time, as well as developmental delays and mobility problems, Oscar has been diagnosed with epilepsy and autism. It was when he received his autism diagnosis that Laura felt she found a community that were dealing with similar kinds of issues as she was. Instagram has been a huge part of her connecting with other parent carers. By sharing aspects of life with Oscar, people have gravitated towards her. She has used the platforms to bring awareness to things like the need for Changing Spaces toilets, the massive underfunding of social services that leaves her with very little respite, and for greater understanding of disabilities in the wider public.

Laura became a single parent while pregnant. During Oscar's first year of life she knew he wasn't developing as he should, and returned again and again to the health visitor and GP, who continually told her she was worrying over nothing. Laura is a nurse and remembers from her days in A&E how they used to have a box to tick called 'worried mother' which is what they would check when they felt sure there was nothing wrong but a mother's high anxiety. The refusal for anyone to acknowledge the issues with Oscar's development, coupled with her own post-natal depression, left Laura feeling alone and doubting herself and her abilities as a mother. Eventually, when he wasn't sitting up, they finally listened and referred her to a developmental paediatrician. With no known reason for Oscar's severe delays, she was never sat down and explained to what to expect, or how things might look in the future. Eventually, nurses started handing her information on services for disabled children and she thought, 'Oh, I suppose I have a disabled child now.' It wasn't a dramatic moment of diagnosis, just a slow realisation that life was starting to look very different for her and Oscar than it did for the mum-friends she had begun to build up around her. Although that friendship group she had made meant a huge amount to her as a single mother, she saw that she was going to need a wider community. As everyone else's children started walking, talking and toilet training, her experiences felt further and further from theirs. That's when the community she created on Instagram started to become a really important part of her life.

Finding a community after more than 30 years as a carer

Valerie Brooks never expected to be a full-time carer to her daughter Jess into adulthood. Jess, who is now 33 and autistic and visually impaired, tried lots of different situations after secondary school, including a day centre, paid carers and also working as a volunteer in an elderly care home. For various reasons – some were not fit for purpose and some made Jess incredibly anxious – none of these ended up working out. Eventually, Valerie made the difficult decision to quit her job as a nurse to be at home with Jess full time. At first Valerie was devastated to stop working in a career she loved. After spending years at home with her children while they were young, Valerie had retrained and begun her career as a nurse; it was never part of her plan to give that up to be back at home again. She also worried what the rest of her family and friends would think, as well as worrying about her future finances. But for Jess's welfare, it was by far the best option that they could come up with so, after years of trying various alternatives, Valerie became a full-time carer.

She decided to start a blog so she could share with friends and family what the two of them were up to, and as a way to process the massive life change that she hadn't planned. A little while after she started blogging, someone stopped her at the supermarket and said how much she was enjoying reading it. She told Valerie that in all the years, she had had no idea what life looked like at home for their family. Other friends and family started saying the same. Valerie's blog grew and so did her Instagram account, which Jess loves making videos for.

When we spoke on the phone, Valerie told me that even though she's now a full-time carer to Jess, she has never felt more connected to her local community and so supported by other carers as she does now. In all the years when Jess was growing up, Valerie had not been sharing her experiences with anyone. They had tried a few support groups, but when they didn't click with the other families, they didn't go back. With school and the various different programmes they had tried, on the surface it must have seemed they had more support. But looking back, Valerie said she didn't have anything like the emotional support she has now. Support that has spilled over from her online accounts into real life meet-ups and connections in her local area. What she had feared so much – the isolation of being a full-time carer and having to retire from a much-loved career – had turned into a positive that she could never have predicted.

Many carers I have spoken to initially started using social media to write and share their experiences as a way to process what they were going through. Almost all of them have been surprised by just how life-changing the emotional support is that comes from online communities. Communities that are there day and night, in your back pocket. It would be easy to underestimate the value of having a community, but it can make a staggering difference to our wellbeing.

The Jo Cox Commission on Loneliness found that the impact of loneliness on physical and mental health is devastating, saying it is as bad for our health as smoking 15 cigarettes a day.[93] Having a supportive community – online and off – can be life-saving in the long run.

Spreading awareness

Emma Terranova, whose mother Jenny has Huntington's disease (see Chapter 5, page 116), spent years forbidden from speaking about the illness with anyone outside of her immediate family. With her mother's consent, in December 2018 Emma set up Campaign For My Brain, a not-for-profit organisation whose aim is to spread awareness of neurological disorders in order to improve the lives of those who have the conditions as well as those who care for them. It has the dual purpose of empowering carers to get the support they need for their loved ones and themselves, as well as bringing public attention to the conditions themselves. Emma says that if there had been less shame and secrecy around her mother's illness when she was a young carer, the situation would have been far more bearable. It was years before she and her sister spoke to anyone at all about their mother. Years spent making excuses to friends and hiding what was happening. Now Emma speaks openly about her life as one of her mother's carers. Forming connections with other families with Huntington's, as well as being able to be open and honest with friends, has been transformative for the family.

Podcasts

It's not just social media that is bringing carers together, podcasts are becoming hubs of community too. Mary Susan McConnell (see Chapter 4, page 93) says each week on her introduction to her Mama Bear podcast that she wants everyone listening to imagine they're sitting on her back porch, enjoying a beverage of their choice and having a conversation with friends. What motivated Mary Susan to begin the podcast was the thought of being with a very sick child in ICU in the middle of the night and feeling so terribly alone. She imagined what it would be like if you could put in your headphones and hear the voices of others who had been through what you're going through.

More than 100 episodes later and she regularly gets messages saying exactly that. That there was no one in their position locally who was going through what they were going through, and the podcast made them feel so much less alone.

Blogs and social media accounts can be wonderful, but there is something so powerful about hearing each other's stories in our own words and voices. Podcasts can also allow for a more nuanced and detailed conversation than the de-contextualised, like-and-share nature of social media. The Mama Bear podcast has episodes on all sorts of topics, and interviews with mothers of kids, from very young to adulthood, who have disabilities of all kinds. Mary Susan has a knack of telling the kinds of stories that show us how much we all have in common, rather than focus on our differences.

The importance of online communities for both carers and those who need support

It can be hard to hear universal cries of the end of civilisation when it comes to social media when you are part of a community that has historically been isolated before the internet gave us access to each other. I look back to my time as a young carer in the 1990s and wonder what life would have been like for me if I had known others who had a parent needing similar support. Would it have made a difference to me if I had known I was not alone? I know it would have made a difference to my mother, who would have been an avid supporter of the mental health campaigners and activists we have today in people such as Matt Haig and Scarlett Curtis. Disabled people have access to communities in a way they never have before thanks to social media, and the same goes for carers. With this increased community comes the ability for disabled people and people who are cared for to tell their own stories, challenge traditional negative narratives and band together to create systemic change. The positives for online communities go far beyond emotional support. They can lead to changes in law and changes in society. Whether because public spaces are so often physically inaccessible, or that poor health means socialising regularly is difficult, or that social communication differences make socialising face to face challenging, the internet has arguably been even more important to disabled people than to non-disabled people. Many carers face similar difficulties of physical isolation, as well as financial barriers to getting out and about regularly.

James Hunt is a single parent to two autistic boys. He co-parents the boys with their mum, who lives close by. When they separated four years ago, it was decided that what the boys needed more than anything was one-to-one support. Jude, now

11, struggled with his younger brother Tommy's noise and outbursts, and keeping them both safe and supported had always been a challenge in the same house. Between them they decided that they would have one of the boys each and swap over every few days, so both boys get to spend time with each parent. It has been fantastic for Tommy and Jude, who experience less anxiety and much needed support from their parents.

While James is thrilled he never has to be apart from either of his boys for too long a period, the relentlessness of single parenting with no breaks takes its toll. James finds it hard to get out in the evenings, especially if one of the boys is going through a particularly tough time. There have been times when they have been through intense periods of anxiety when even their grandparents have struggled to look after them for an evening. Both boys find it hard to cope being around lots of people, so socialising at weekends with friends is often not possible, or only for very short amounts of time. Over the years it has meant James, who works from home, can go long periods without spending time with another adult. This is a common scenario for many carers who are caring full time for someone completely dependent on them for all their needs. When socialising is out of the reach of the disabled or ill person you are supporting, then that can mean it's out of reach for the carer too.

James started a blog that has become his connection to his family and friends as well as other parent carers. He tells me that isolation is one of the hardest things about their situation. He doesn't want to force the boys to socialise at the weekends because he knows it can be too distressing for them, but it can lead to him feeling very alone at times. What started as a blog has grown into a large community on social media, a podcast and now in-person meet-ups for families raising autistic kids.

Online abuse

While the benefits of social media are arguably very large for disabled people, people with chronic illnesses and those who support loved ones, the downsides can also be great. In May 2019 UK charity Leonard Cheshire reported that between 2017 and 2018 there was a 33% rise in online hate crime against disabled people.[94] The kind of abuse that disabled people experience online is wide, and includes images of people with visible disabilities (particularly children) being used to make memes and jokes, being told they're better off dead or should have been aborted, and being targeted for 'miracle cures'. People with learning difficulties are targeted for exploitation, people with visible disabilities mocked for the way they look, and people with invisible disabilities being told they are faking or can't be disabled.[95] The horrific list of offences goes on. A Parliamentary Committee investigating online abuse in January 2019 heard from many campaigners, charities and disabled people that this online abuse is a symptom of the wider problem of how disability is viewed in society and that social media has intensified and normalised this abuse. But the benefits to being online are far too great to the disabled community to simply 'shut down' social media as many, far more privileged people are suggesting.

Jaron Lanier, author of *Ten Arguments For Deleting Your Social Media Accounts Right Now*, writes that it is not the internet that is the necessarily the problem, but the algorithms based on business models that aim to change our behaviour in order to benefit the customer. We are not the customer, all the brands vying for our attention are. We are the product. In this current scenario, Lanier argues that we are all prone to becoming trolls and assholes.[96] Deleting accounts might be suitable for many people who have access to socialising and activism in other ways

– people whose stories are already reflected in mainstream media. For those who are in minorities or are socially or physically isolated, social media has become too powerful a tool to give up just because of backlash and abuse.

In-person connection

While social media is a fantastic way to find and connect with others whose circumstances reflect our own, wherever possible bringing those connections into face-to-face meet-ups is well worth the effort it can take. Tanya Savva (see Chapter 2, page 57) had been in a unique position as both a parent of a disabled child and an occupational therapist working with other families with disabled children. What became clear to her was that unless the parents were well supported, their children were not going to thrive. When she put up a post on Facebook to gauge interest in an in-person retreat to support mothers of disabled and chronically ill children, it turned out to receive the most traffic of any post she had written.

She planned the first retreat meticulously, with a timetable packed with activities. But when the attendees arrived, something far more magical happened. She realised what every woman there needed was connection. Tanya found herself stepping back and just allowing the connections to happen, and ended up halving the content of the weekend. She told me that for many of the women it was the first time they had felt seen and heard in a long time, as well as feeling free to share some of their darkest thoughts about the difficulties they had been through. Many had arrived exhausted and not knowing how they would continue – and left feeling buoyed up and supported by the group. The women who had come for the long weekend retreat had all been strangers when they arrived and they left as close friends, staying in touch and continuing to support each other long after the retreat had finished.

While a retreat might be out of reach for most of us, connecting is something we all need. As mentioned already, loneliness is much higher in carers than in the general population. In the US, one mother of a disabled child has started an app called Wolf and Friends, which pairs people with other parent carers in the area. Facebook groups, podcasts and Instagram accounts spill offline and into local meet-ups, swapped phone numbers and private WhatsApp groups. But as much as we need other people in a similar situation to ourselves, we also need a community of friends and family around us, and often we need paid support as well.

Learning to ask for help

As a young carer, I had learned to look after myself at an early age. This continued as I went off to school, travelled independently and eventually moved to London. By the time my mother died, though I was devastated, I had not been accustomed to being looked after by her in a very long time. Independence had always paid off for me.

With the arrival of my daughter along with Arthur's high needs, all of that self-reliance came crashing down around me. As much as I desperately wished I could do it all on my own, I realised that it was no longer going to be possible. Although I have always had strong relationships with friends, I realised I had been priding myself on not relying on any of them. When I needed help, I found that it was too painful and made me feel too vulnerable to ask. But for Arthur's sake, especially when my marriage was over, I was going to have to learn how.

When we divorced, Arthur and Agnes' father and I decided it was best if Arthur always stayed in the family home for the time being. So every other weekend, their father arrives to spend time with them, and I leave. This has been a great decision for both children, and has made what could have been a huge disruption much smoother. But it has also meant that over the years I have had to stay with friends, ask favours and be in other people's spaces rather than my own. It has not always been comfortable to ask for this help, but without family in this country and with Arthur's needs being what they are, it has been necessary. Learning to rely on those around me has turned out to be one of the most humbling and beneficial side effects of being a single parent and a motherless mother. But I would have to fall to my knees before I figured this out.

The ups and downs of paid support

Though paid help has been essential to me continuing to work, over the years I have had my fair share of unreliable help. Understandably, when you pay someone to support your family, it's simply a job to them and the rest of their life must come first. I've had brilliant nannies leave London, get pregnant or become unwell. I have had mediocre ones call in sick over and over again, including one who simply disappeared one day without a trace. The hardest one of all, though, was when a new promising carer quit after two weeks. She confessed that she found it too difficult to manage Arthur and would cry at home every night after work. The night she told me I sat on the kitchen floor and howled. All the careful planning and interviewing to get the right support will never prepare you for the moment someone tells you they can't manage to do for 20 hours a week what you are doing alone, for years on end. It's enough to make you never want to trust anyone again.

But each time I have had to pick myself up and get on with life because I have no choice. I have a child who can't attend after-school clubs or holiday clubs or go to friends' houses to play. A child whose schedule is decided by when the local authority bus picks him up and drops him off each day, something I have no control over. For those of us combining caring with paid work, this is one of the hardest aspects.

In all the mess and chaos of being let down by paid carers, I discovered something so important. Though my friends have busy lives, they will always be willing to step up in an emergency. I have been stuck on photoshoots across town and got messages from a nanny saying they won't be there to meet the school bus that day because they're too ill, and friends have dropped everything to step in. I have taken my daughter to A&E with an asthma attack many times, and friends have left their own children with neighbours in order to be at home with Arthur to save him the distress of having to come to their house. When I couldn't figure out how to take my kids on holiday alone when Arthur needed so much support from me, friends have come away with us.

There is much about being a carer that forces you to let go of your ego. I never would have asked for help from friends unless I was forced to, and our relationships have become so much closer for it. Friends have told me it feels good to know the ways in which they can be helpful, just as it feels good for me to know how I can be helpful to them in return. As I have had to let my walls crumble, I noticed that in refusing to ask for help in the past I had been judgmental of those who appeared to need so much support – that inner pride, born from necessity but kept up as a barrier to being vulnerable to being let down, as my mother had often let me down. But if I had never been forced to ask for and accept the support of others, I would never have truly known how deep our friendships ran. Like Marisa coming with me to take my mother to a psychiatric ward, my London friends have picked me up and dusted me off and allowed me to join in life in a way that I could never do had I clung to independence.

It is hard to reach out for help. It's especially hard in a culture where everyone is busy and we are praised for doing it all and doing it on our own. It is vital that as carers we reject this idea of hyper-independence, because we cannot and should not do this alone. Though many of the carers I have spoken to receive financial support towards paid carers, this only solves part of the problem. Some receive enough to help pay for support for their loved one, but cannot find good-quality carers in the area willing to do the work for the money they are allowed to pay. Others find the best paid carers move on quickly, leaving them continually searching for new ones. Paid carers can call in sick, leaving us holding the fort, no matter what our other commitments might have been that day. Paid carers must be managed like any other staff: training them, doing payroll and other admin, which is time-consuming and adds to the workload.

Paid carers, though essential for many of us, bring a huge amount of extra work and stress. Here are just a few of the stories that carers shared about the difficulty of relying on paid care. Each morning Claire Kotecha, whose son Anand has night nurses every night (see Chapter 2, page 61), has to complete an official change-over from the night nurse to herself, to the nurse who accompanies Anand to school. This means she struggles to spend any time with either of her children in the morning; she's simply too busy managing medical staff. Ruth and Steve (see Chapter 3, page 79), after Steve's spinal injury, have managed pretty well just the two of them, but when Steve's health has gone through a bad patch, they have been offered only some paid support in the form of a carer for Steve. Neither of them want a paid carer for Steve; what they need is support around the house so that Ruth can be the one supporting Steve when he needs it. But that kind of help is just not available to them.

Laura Moore, whose son William has cerebral palsy, has enough hours of paid carer funds from social services for what they need as a family, but finds it impossible to find good-quality carers in their area. Lots of the money allocated to William goes unspent and is sent back to the Local Authority, even though Laura would desperately love to be able to use it. Many carers spend huge amounts of time chasing paid carers who fail to turn up, finding emergency cover when someone calls in sick, or simply having to drop other responsibilities when they are let down.

Paid carers are essential for so many, but it can feel risky and exposing to have to rely on them. Many people I spoke to would rather do everything themselves if they could. With the social-care system buckling under the weight of ten years' of worth of government cuts, there is simply not enough money to go around. At the moment everyone – including those who have terminal illness, life-long, untreatable conditions and progressive conditions with no chance of recovery – is forced into being continually re-assessed for their eligibility for social care. These assessments can be invasive and extremely stressful for both the person who needs care and their family members. Many people will let themselves become burned out administering the care themselves rather than rely on social care that can be taken away at any time.

It can also be difficult when the person you are supporting doesn't want to be helped by people outside of their family. Many carers put off applying for social care for a long time, knowing their partner or parent is resistant to the idea. Sometimes they have burned themselves out long before they finally ask for outside help.

Paid carers from agencies who provide daily support with personal care needs such as getting someone out of bed and dressing them, are often on such tight schedules before their next appointment that they must rush through the process, taking no account of the preferences and emotional needs of the person they're attending to. This has become a progressively worse problem for disabled, chronically ill and elderly people over the last few years. Many working-age disabled people have been forced out of independent living and into completely inappropriate group homes, after successfully living independently with the right kind of support for years.[97]

Managing paid support if and when we can afford it or get allocated it, can be extremely stressful, but is a vital part of expanding our community when we have someone else so dependent on us. Jess Wilson (see Chapter 3, page 74) told me that it was an autistic friend of hers who pointed out to her the vital need for expanding her daughter Brooke's network of support beyond immediate family, and to include paid support. She reminded her that it was pretty blinkered to believe that a parent was the only one who could support a disabled child's needs. Parents don't live forever. Parents get burnout and can become a danger to their children when they do so. Jess admitted to me that expanding Brooke's support network is something she is still trying to work on, but she was grateful to her friend for reminding her that creating a circle of support is not selfish, but in fact the opposite, avoiding putting the person you support at risk.

We need many kinds of communities

Our communities are made up of no single one thing. We need friends who understand and have lived experience of what we are going through, who can listen without judgment and without attempting to 'fix' our situations. We need family and friends who step in and offer help when they can, who can become our back-up for when things go wrong and emergencies occur. Who simply remember to keep checking in on us and inviting us out, even if we can rarely say yes. Who are willing to adjust gatherings to make them accessible to our disabled family members, without us having to constantly remind everyone what those needs are.

We need schools and other institutions who make us and our disabled family members feel welcome, understood and of value. We need paid support in order to help us get sleep, eat, earn a living and recharge. Eventually many of us will need communities who will take over the care of our loved ones when we no longer can. We need so much from others and that is not easy to admit in this cultural climate when we are expected to be 'enough' all on our own. But humans are never supposed to do this alone. We are a species that thrives when we are in communities that support us and hold us and care for us.

Twenty years on from my mother's death, Marisa is still my best friend. She is the first one I call when things go wrong as well as when things go right. It feels as though friendships forged during times when you are so vulnerable and so in need have a way of lasting long distances, and major life changes. Over the years I have come to rely on many wonderful friends who have rescued me when paid help falls through, and who have continually stepped in to share holidays and help out wherever they can. I have been incredibly lucky in friendship in my life. But unless I needed this help, unless I had been forced to not be an island, determined to do things myself, I would never have known the kind of support that is possible between friends. Being a carer has allowed me to learn to rely on others, and I'm so grateful for all the love it has shown me.

CHAPTER 9

Purpose

'What I've come to see is not that things happen for a reason, but there is some sort of trick whereby you can look at your mangled wreckage and from it craft meaning and purpose.'[98]

Cathy Rentzenbrink, author

Emma Terranova (see Chapter 5, page 116) was a teenager when she decided she would have to become a nurse. With her mother already experiencing symptoms of Huntington's disease, she knew it was her best chance to be able to support and advocate for her. But after a frightening choking incident, Emma changed her mind. Nursing training would make her a good carer, but being a paramedic could save her life. She chose the latter and was pleased to discover it was well suited to her. She was a working paramedic by the age of 21 and, though young, she already had more life experience with disability and mental illness than many of her colleagues. She could recognise and deal patiently with the confusion and frustrations of people with brain injuries and neurological conditions. She was not afraid or judgmental of addicts and those with severe mental illnesses.

Emma says her colleagues sometimes get frustrated when it becomes clear that a call-out wasn't 100% necessary. But Emma knows what it's like to be a carer and scared. So often those calls are from carers who are afraid and don't want to be alone as their loved one has an episode, or is dying – even when it's expected and planned for, even when medication and instructions are on hand. Emma knows how frightening it can be to be a carer and be entirely responsible for another human who is so vulnerable. She also understands how frightening it is for her mother to be confused and unable to communicate her needs, and that it's not her fault that she lashes out. Being a paramedic has given Emma the medical knowledge to speak up for her mother and fight for her needs to be met. It means she can calmly deal with a choking incident and can administer medication with confidence. But more than that, Emma is certain being a carer is the reason she is so good at her job.

Our roles as carers, whether they happen very suddenly or gradually over time, can change who we are and how we interact with the world. While many of us gain a great sense of purpose through the act of caring itself, others find that the role opens their eyes to a whole new sense of purpose. Whether it's the desire to protect a loved one, as in Emma's case, or not being able to un-see the great injustices facing disabled people around the world, to needing to find something outside of the home to focus on – spending a lot of time supporting someone else can help us to recognise what is most important to us.

In Japan there is a term which sums up neatly this sense of purpose seen in many carers: *ikigai*, or a reason for being. Ikigai is credited as one of the aspects for the long and healthy life spans of the people of Hokkaido, one of the world's 'blue zones' where residents regularly live past 100. Ikigai is often illustrated as a Venn diagram of four intersecting circles. The circles represent what you are good at, what you love, what the world needs and what would earn an income. In the centre where these four circles intersect is the place we will find our *ikigai*. Rick Hanson, in his book *Resilient*, refers to a similar intersection of three qualities: likes, talents and values.[99] Hanson writes that to honour your dreams is an important aspect of leading a resilient life. And resilience is something we all need in our lives as carers.

When advocacy forces you out of hiding

When Natalie Weaver was 34 weeks pregnant, she was told that her baby daughter would have face, hand and feet deformities. Without a solid reason as to why, the doctors weren't sure if her condition was life-threatening and whether she would survive the birth. But Sophia did survive, and though she went on to have multiple surgeries, she made it home. Aside from the complex medical difficulties, Natalie soon discovered there was a whole other aspect to being Sophia's mother to deal with. People were made very uncomfortable with Sophia's facial differences, and when she took her out, kids would sometimes point, or even on occasion scream; adults would often either stare or turn away in avoidance, crossing the street to get away from them. 'It broke me. It was a pain that brought me to my knees,' she told me. At first Natalie tried to hide her feelings of sadness and pretend to family and friends that the reactions of strangers didn't bother her. But she was deeply bothered. She would take days and even weeks to recover from trips out. 'I would have to build up courage and strength and be in the best place possible, just to go to the grocery store with my child.'

Natalie kept trying to get Sophia out and about so she could experience what other children could, but it became more and more difficult as they faced so much discrimination and hatred. She tells me if it had been discrimination against herself it would have been bad enough, but to witness your own child being rejected in that way was devastating. When Sophia was around three years old, it became clear that as well as Rett syndrome, a degenerative genetic condition that includes muscle spasticity, regression of skills, breathing irregularity and seizures, she also had severe problems with her immune system. This meant that she was no longer able to go out in public – where risks of infections were high – especially as her facial differences meant her mouth didn't fully close, leaving her vulnerable to germs. Natalie said it was a legitimate excuse for them to retreat from the world. They were a private family, who behind closed doors vowed to shower Sophia with as much unconditional love, adoration and fun as was humanly possible.

When Sophia was seven years old the access to healthcare for disabled children that wasn't covered by private insurance in North Carolina, where the Weavers live, came under threat. This healthcare is absolutely vital to the lives of disabled children, as private insurance doesn't cover medical equipment or wheelchairs, and it doesn't cover any social care or nursing care at home. When she found out that the services provided were going to be cut by 70%, Natalie realised in that moment that she had to do something to protect Sophia's and other children's access to healthcare. She decided after years of fierce privacy to share their story in the media. She joined some other parent carers to form an organisation called Advocates for Medically Fragile Kids NC and, within six weeks, they successfully prevented the cuts from happening. Natalie had always been a strong private advocate for Sophia but now she realised that she could take that further, to support the rights of disabled and chronically ill people beyond her own family.

The first time Natalie wrote and delivered a speech of any kind, she was flown to Washington, D.C. to speak at a press conference in front of five senators. Sophia and Natalie's story went viral and she became a loud voice in the fight to protect disabled people's access to healthcare. As she built up supporters for their cause, it came with a lot of abuse. She had expected some, after her earlier experiences had shown her, but it was on a scale she was unprepared for. People told her she should kill her daughter, that she was a drain on society, and all sorts of insults were made about her appearance. This time, with access to healthcare at risk, the stakes were too high to just disappear in fear again. Natalie decided to withstand the online abuse, knowing she could shield her daughter from it at least. But then it went too far.

In 2017 a man used an image of Sophia to promote eugenics on Twitter, and when she contacted Twitter to have the post taken down, she discovered there was no way to report someone for the abuse of disabled people on the platform. You could report someone for inciting racial, religious or gender-based hatred but you could not do the same for disabled people, a group that experiences some of the highest levels of abuse on social media. Within days of campaigning heavily via traditional and social media, Twitter listened, and included discrimination against disabled people, in the form of hate speech and harassment, in their reporting tool. It was at this point that Natalie realised that her work as an advocate needed to go far beyond access to healthcare. If she was to be a good ally to people like her daughter, she would have to advocate for her daughter's right to exist in public spaces without being vulnerable to abuse. She had found a purpose.

Seeing through a new lens

The act of supporting a family member can also cause a shift in focus around a career that already existed. Vaila Morrison was working as an architect designing homes and housing extensions when she gave birth to her first child. But when it became apparent that her daughter Elidh had an unknown genetic disorder that was causing severe developmental delays, Vaila wasn't able to return to work and meet her needs at the same time. As time went by it became clear that Elidh would always have limited mobility and an intellectual disability, requiring support for life. Vaila started the process of making adaptations to their house for it to be fully accessible, and as she dove into the project, she found it overwhelming, with information about accessible builds and applying for grants extremely hard to come by and very confusing, even with her training. She started to blog about her experiences, sharing information with other families who needed an accessible home but didn't know where to begin. Her research led her to some pretty stark conclusions. She realised that though accessibility is given a nod in most sustainable design, with an ageing population, and the needs of a family changing across a lifetime, a building could never be considered sustainable unless it was fully inclusive. Inclusive design, she says, is not a niche. When we design for the people who have the greatest accessibility needs, we make environments that are more accessible to everyone.

Vaila now campaigns on many issues around housing, including the idea that just as we now consider energy efficiency when we renovate our older homes, we should also be considering inclusive design, even when there is currently no disabled person living in the house. Vaila is also campaigning to make new multi-home developments meet the Lifetime Homes Standard as a minimum requirement.

Vaila believes that all designers have an obligation to consider the needs of all sorts of people who might be accessing the place, including friends and family who will visit, but also when a family may have periods of time pushing babies in buggies and when inevitably our needs change as we age. Inclusive design is far more than wheelchair accessible and ugly plastic grab rails, she told me. If we are to have a society that values and welcomes disabled people into public and private spaces, we need to see beautiful and exciting inclusive design in the mainstream. Alongside her campaigning, her blog and Instagram account is filled with inexpensive and fun adaptations for families with the hashtag inclusivechic. Her dream, she says, is to see inclusive design become everyday design.

Vaila has spent a lot of time campaigning for more Changing Places toilets. Specifically she wants to see them included as a part of building regulations for new builds that service large numbers of the public. Currently there is no legal obligation to provide anything more than an accessible toilet, which for many disabled people will not be accessible at all. If a person is using a large electric wheelchair, needs assistance moving from their chair with a carer or is incontinent, then traditional accessible toilets are not fit for purpose.

A reason to get out of bed

Much has been written about our need as humans for purpose and meaning. We all need a reason to get out of bed in the morning. There are now many studies that point to a sense of purpose as a strong reason for people's resilience in the face of adversity, and the ability to get up when they are knocked down by failure, setbacks and trauma.

Natalie Weaver initially found purpose in being the best mother and carer to Sophia that she could be. She also retreated from the world and hid away, not just to protect her daughter but to protect her own heart too. But she realised that this retreat from the world was not sustainable. She needed a wider purpose to make it possible to face the difficulties of the outside world. That purpose has grown and grown. Natalie is now the founder of Sophia's Voice, a charity that raises awareness for children with disabilities and facial differences, as well as raising money for families in medical debt and who need vital medical equipment that they can't afford. Sophia was very much a part of the organisation. Though she was non-speaking, she was able to communicate in other ways and, together with her mother, made decisions that steered the mission and direction of the charity. It was a project they worked on together until Sophia's death in May 2019. Natalie has continued the work since then, in line with both her and her daughter's values.

Carers are often pushed out of the traditional working world. Many find it impossible to meet the demands of a full-time job alongside their caring responsibilities. Employers are often inflexible, unable to make allowances for time off for medical appointments, or the need to work from home sometimes when the person being supported goes through periods of poor health. Among the carers I have come into contact with, many have left professions in the NHS and teaching. These front-line services are often the most inflexible kinds of work, despite the fact that the personal experiences that a carer has can add enormously to these environments. Mothers of disabled children in particular find it difficult to work, with much of the unpaid caring foisted on their shoulders. Along with the caring, there are large amounts of admin that go into getting a disabled child access to education, which often require many hours of advocacy work and, in lots of cases, tribunal appearances and appeals that can go on for years.

Natalie Lee was a midwife working for the NHS when her eldest daughter was born. By the time she had another child, she could see her shift work was unsustainable, with the needs of her daughter – who was losing her sight – along with the usual demands of family life. Natalie started blogging about another passion of hers, fashion. Within a few years she had a large following and was making her income flexibly as an influencer and fashion blogger, focusing on intersectional feminism and body image. When her husband completed the Three Peaks challenge in aid of The Royal Society for Blind Children (RSBC) and raised over £25,000, the charity approached Natalie and asked her if she'd like to become an ambassador. Natalie hadn't really used her platform much to discuss her daughter's disability at this point, but when she looked into the statistics around employment for blind working-age adults, she was shocked. 90% of blind adults are unable to find work due to employers being unwilling to make adaptations to the work environment or because of direct discrimination. Natalie realised that becoming an ambassador and sharing her family's story with a wide audience could help change society's views of visual impairment, improving the lives of those working-age adults who need work opportunities.

The skills gained as an advocate for the person you are supporting can hugely benefit the workplace. Leanne Patrick went back to university to get a nursing degree after her youngest daughter, who is autistic and has learning difficulties, went to pre-school. She was only able to do so because her husband Ali worked part time and from home. Leanne has gone on to specialise in mental health and is currently doing her masters. When we spoke she said that Ella is a big influence on how active she has become in student nursing politics and in her approach as a nurse.

It can take effort and ingenuity to continue working when you have someone very dependent on you, and even then it's not always possible. Laura Godfrey (see Chapter 8, page 191) is a single parent and is unable to return to work as an NHS nurse. The childcare just isn't available for Oscar's high needs, and shift work requires long days. She would love to return to work and her experience as a carer to someone with epilepsy, autism and learning difficulties would be of value in her work environment. The NHS has a poor track record with learning difficulties, which is finally being acknowledged (see Chapter 3, page 90). But with people like Laura, willing but unable to get back into inflexible hospital shift work, it's hard to see how attitudes and understanding will change within the NHS anytime soon.

All of these carers have something in common. They have taken their experiences within their own families and are using the skills and knowledge they have gained to act in service of others. This is how many people turn challenging and life-changing circumstances around and find a sense of meaning and purpose in situations that are beyond their control. In her book *The Power of Meaning*, Emily Esfahani Smith describes the problems with our current obsession with happiness in modern society. While we may live relatively comfortable lives, the wealthiest countries in the world are experiencing record levels of suicide, depression and anxiety. Countries like Denmark paradoxically report both high rates of happiness and high rates of suicide. While there are some theories that this might be partly due to the extra difficulties of being an unhappy person in a largely happy country, Emily Esfahani Smith has found another reason. If you have plenty of happiness you may have a life of comfort and ease, but if it lacks meaning it will simply not be enough to lead a fulfilling life.[100] She writes that as the happiness industry has grown exponentially over the last couple of decades, as a society we are more miserable than ever. Social scientists have uncovered yet another paradox, one that author Ruth Whippman also explores in her recent book *The Pursuit of Happiness*. Chasing feelings of happiness makes us unhappy.[101]

Though positive psychology is well known for its research into happiness, its larger mission is to explore how people can lead deep and fulfilling lives. Martin Seligman, one of the pioneers of positive psychology, called a meaningful life one in which you use your strengths to serve others. When we are thrown into challenging situations, we often uncover strengths we had no idea we possessed – and cultivate others that we have never had to use before. For Natalie Weaver that meant taking the confidence she had advocating for Sophia and applying it to a wider community of disabled children. For Vaila it was using her knowledge of architecture and building regulations to campaign for more accessible housing and toilets.

In her book, Emily Esfahani Smith says that psychologists have found that when people describe their lives as meaningful, they have met three conditions. They evaluate their lives as having been significant and part of something bigger, they think their lives make sense, and they are driven by a strong sense of purpose. In a study conducted by Florida State University,[102] it was found that people who lead lives that they described as meaningful may have had more moments of feeling anxious and stressed and fewer moments of positive feelings like ease and pleasure, but they also felt more connected to others and as though they were contributing to something larger than themselves. The most common example of this is having children, which is well known to correlate with lower levels of happiness day to day but higher levels of purpose overall.

In a 2010 study,[103] university students were split into two groups, where one group was asked to perform an act of hedonia (pleasure) for themselves each day, while the other group was asked to perform an act of eudomonia (meaning). Amongst the meaningful acts were forgiving a friend, studying, or helping another person. In the pleasure group, activities that they reported doing were things like playing a game, going shopping and eating sweets. At the end of the study the students in the pleasure group had experienced more positive, happy feelings during and immediately after the study than the students in the meaning group. But three months later, those feelings had worn off. In the meaning group, however, three months later they reported fewer negative moods than the pleasure group and were more likely to say they felt part of something larger than themselves.

A couple of years ago, Vicki, whose eldest child Jimmy is autistic, was becoming very frustrated with the effort it was taking to get out and about with her family. She would go to a quiet hour at their local soft play centre, only to be asked by another parent of a disabled child if she had managed to get to a rare local autism-friendly event the weekend before, yet she had never seen it advertised anywhere. Vicki started searching and couldn't find any central point at all that listed events, workshops, special openings and quiet hours designed to be accessible to families with a disabled family member. The only websites she could find focused on wheelchair accessibility, which though incredibly important, didn't provide the information she needed. Frustrated and fed up with the intense amounts of research that went into each outing, she decided to build the resource herself, and Hard Days Out was born. With the help of families all over the UK, Vicki has built a website that lists museums, galleries, city farms, National Trust properties and all sorts of days out and one-off events. The aim of Hard Days Out is to take some of the guesswork and time-consuming research out of figuring out whether a place would be suitable for your family to visit.

Vicki told me that most organisations only list wheelchair access and disabled parking on their websites, forgetting to add all sorts of other information that might be essential to those with a family member with more complex needs. When she started digging, she realised that often larger organisations had fantastic services that they didn't bother to advertise, even on their own social media outlets. How can a place claim to be disability friendly, she told me, if they aren't even letting families know what is on offer for them? Vicki started thinking about all the questions she needed answered before she could decide whether it would be accessible for her family. Is it an open space or are there gates? Are there lots of dogs off leads? Do you need to bring ID and proof of disability to access the free carer entrance ticket? What equipment is in the playground and what times of day is it busiest? Are the staff helpful and understand what help you need? I found myself nodding along with her. All these are questions that many organisations don't realise can be essential in assessing whether a disabled or chronically ill person will be able to access and enjoy an experience.

As Vicki began to build up the resources on the website, she could see a desperate need for these places to better understand the needs of families like hers, if they really wanted to serve whole communities. As a secondary school teacher with many years' experience, she realised she could use her teaching skills to put together workshops for companies and organisations who were willing to improve their accessibility. It was one thing to have plenty of reviews on the website, but if most of the places had a poor understanding of what families wanted and needed from a day out, it was going to be of little use. Hard Days Out inclusion consultancy began, and now Vicki – who is also completing a post graduate diploma in autism studies – is delivering workshops to all kinds of organisations, big and small, on how to make themselves more accessible.

Vicki said that most places want to improve but worry about the extra costs of providing for all kinds of families. Retrofitting an old building with a Changing Places toilet might be out of reach for many small businesses, but there are so many small things that can be done that cost relatively little but can make a big difference to how welcoming a place is. Vicki feels the impact she is having with Hard Days Out is even greater than her work as a part-time teacher. With the resources and the consultancy, she is able to have a direct impact on the lives of so many families like her own. And it feels good to be of service to others.

When we can create positive and purposeful action out of difficult experiences, we can begin to make sense of them. And making sense of our lives is an important part of finding meaning. Emily Esfahani Smith writes that one of the other pillars of a meaningful life is storytelling. When we can tell our stories in coherent ways that make sense of what we have experienced, and reframe our lives to include purpose, we are far more resilient. Just as the study that showed writing about our traumas helps us to process them and make sense of them, the stories we tell about ourselves and our lives can help us see ourselves in a more meaningful light. Years after my experiences supporting my mother, I can see that those early lessons have had a positive impact on my ability to cope with the extra challenges of raising a disabled child. While I'd happily give back those lessons in exchange for my mother, that, unfortunately, isn't possible. So I'll gladly accept my consolation prize in the hopes that it has made me a more compassionate mother to Arthur.

Service

It's not just in work that carers find a sense of purpose. Many find that although caring can be difficult at times, it can bring a great sense of purpose through being of service to someone you love. Some people find that although they may at times be resentful or sad, this sense of purpose helps to carry them through. Others find that after their loved one has died, there is a strong feeling of pride for having been the person who supported a beloved family member through difficult times.

This is not straightforward. It can take time to figure out *how* best to be of service to the person who needs you. When Emma and Kelly Terranova (see Chapter 5, page 116) were told of their mother Jenny's Huntington's diagnosis as teenagers, Kelly was heading off to university, and so the role of caregiver naturally fell to Emma, who was still living at home. Over the years, Kelly has struggled to give as much hands-on support to her mother as Emma. She has felt a huge lack of confidence in contrast to her sister's capable and medically trained hands. She spent many years avoiding hands-on caring for her mother, afraid of seeing her mother's decline up close, angry at the unfairness of the disease, and scared of the possibility she too would carry the same gene and have the same fate.

With her father and her sister carrying out the majority of the care, Kelly found herself looking for other ways to contribute. She began a huge fundraising project which raised a large amount of money for a charity aimed at finding effective treatments and cures. Together with a friend they have made a documentary with the purpose of raising awareness of Huntington's, to improve the lives of those living with it, as well as those who care for them.

As Jenny's disease has progressed, Kelly has had to step up

even more to support her father and sister. But caring for her mother still makes her feel very anxious. She misses the feeling of being cared for by her mother deeply, and doing the hands-on practical caring is a sharp reminder of that loss. Counselling has helped her to understand that much of the anger and anxiety is grief. Just knowing that, she says, has been a huge help.

In every family experiencing the difficulties of supporting a loved one, different people will occupy different roles. Kelly says: 'I often feel like the weak link in our family and I worry I've let Mum down. On days like this I just try to remember none of us choose this situation.' Kelly has found that when the act of caring has felt overwhelming, raising awareness and money to help find a cure has been her way of finding a sense of purpose in her mother's illness.

Grace is a single mother to 12-year-old Ami. Ami is medically complex, with a diagnosis of cerebral palsy, hydrocephalus, lung disease, seizures and visual and hearing impairments, amongst many others. Since she was born early at just 25 weeks, Ami has had at least one life-threatening episode each year of her life. In the early years, Grace told me she found herself obsessing unhealthily over cleanliness, desperate to keep her daughter's health as good as possible. She fought hard to provide her daughter with the advocacy she needed, as well as lots of enriching experiences for her. Grace never stopped.

Then about six years ago, her own health went into decline. She assumed she was getting burned out and thought all she needed was a bit more rest. But months and months went by with no change. Her GP told her she must be depressed, but she didn't feel depressed. Grace was physically exhausted all the time and had a whole host of other symptoms, including severe back pain. Eventually, she was diagnosed with ME (Chronic Fatigue Syndrome), as well as an autoimmune condition affecting her thyroid, endometriosis and damage to her spine, likely caused by her caring responsibilities. Grace had to cut everything back. Struggling to socialise as it was with Ami's high needs, she found many friends fell away when she didn't recover quickly. Any chance she had of going back to work, which was already going to be challenging with Ami's needs, went completely out of the window.

What at first was a terrible low point in her life turned out to be a huge turning point for Grace. She was forced to slow down. As she slowed down and learned to accept she couldn't control everything, she started to relax a little. Each time Ami faced a life-threatening episode, Grace found herself asking, how do I want to be if this is her last day? She knew what the answer was. She wanted Ami to experience as much love and care as possible. That became Grace's purpose.

Grace let go of the friends who weren't understanding, and of a romantic relationship too. She began an Instagram account with her daughter that shares Ami's incredible exuberance for life, even though it is more physically restricted than many. Every now and again, when Grace is filling out paperwork for a yearly review or going through Ami's paperwork with a new doctor, she says she is overwhelmed by what she sees on paper. Ami should not be alive, Grace told me. She is a strong and resilient girl who, looking at her list of complex needs, should not be here. Grace says that this reminds her that she is fulfilling her purpose every day. She has managed to keep her daughter alive longer than anyone imagined possible. It is in this act of service for Ami that Grace has felt her most fulfilled.

Grace doesn't discuss her own chronic illnesses very much. She doesn't like to dwell on the difficulties that Ami faces either. She said that her own illness was instrumental in questioning how she wanted to live the limited time she has with her daughter. And for Grace that means not dwelling on the hard stuff. At any point Ami could have a seizure, or contract a chest infection, or dislodge the shunt in her brain and that could be the end of her life. Grace tries to treat every day as if it were Ami's last, wanting her interaction with Ami and Ami's interactions with the world to be as positive as possible. She has chosen to tell her story, as one of service, gratitude and joy, even among some of the extreme difficulties they experience. For many of us who have not experienced the difficulties involved in supporting a child, partner or parent through a life-limiting condition, it may seem impossible that life could be seen through such a positive and joyful lens. But as you'll see from the next chapter, there is much we can learn from the many carers who do.

CHAPTER 10

Joy

'Joy comes in sips, not gulps.'

Sharon Draper, author and educator

I have an old video on my phone that we all like to watch sometimes. Arthur is two years old and we are at a friend's house who hosted a music group for us each week. Arthur had never engaged with group activities at this point; none of them had seemed to hold his interest at all. Storytelling was out, he was only interested if it was one his favourite books to read one-on-one to him. He didn't follow movements or show interest in what other children were doing, and he was always driven by internal desires and interests that were often nothing to do with what was on offer. I didn't mind. I found it strange in a way, when children were cajoled into group activities, their play led by someone else. It felt ok to just let Arthur do his own thing. I signed up for the music class because after the first session I could see *some* of it was going to be interesting to him. He would move about the room, climbing and doing his own thing while the musician would tell stories using instruments, allowing the kids to call out answers to questions.

That held no interest at all to Arthur. But these sessions were run by incredible young musicians, Royal Academy graduates who were bumping up their income by working with toddlers and pre-schoolers on weekday mornings. So a time would come when they would sit down at the keyboard and play Mozart, Chopin or Vivaldi. This was Arthur's favourite part. He would twirl and dance and squeal with delight. The other children enjoyed it too, of course, but watching these videos it is obvious to everyone that the level of excitement and intense sensory experience that Arthur was feeling was on a whole different level. He is loud, listening hard and moving incessantly. Arthur has always experienced everything on another level. While this can mean meltdowns, overwhelm and anxiety, it also means euphoric joy in small and seemingly insignificant experiences.

It is through Arthur that I have seen how much we intellectualise joy and pleasurable experiences. Our focus on what will make us happy can lead us to be driven into planning ahead, spending money, worrying and anticipating. And yet so often this creates a pressure that can lead to disappointment afterwards. Did the experience meet our expectations? Was it all we hoped for? As a parent to a child who does not conform to expected behaviour or interaction with the world around, it has made me question how I find my own sense of pleasure in the world. A question I probably could have easily avoided if both my children had developed typically.

How do we find fun when our life has many restrictions?

Our life can be more restricted in some ways then other families. It can take a huge amount of planning for us to take part in activities that other families can do on a whim, and it would be quite easy to get caught up in the difficulty of it all. An activity might be desperately desired by my daughter but completely unsuitable for my son. It's not always a matter of having enough helping hands either. So often it's just of no interest to Arthur, and to drag him along for the sake of inclusion and for *doing things as a family*, just because that's what everyone else does, would be to the detriment of all of us. So everything we do must be questioned. Is it worth it? What will Arthur gain from it? Will the struggles be worth it for the moments of pleasure and the potential expansion of our world? Can I manage the situation or will I run myself into exhaustion if I try it? Or do we divide and conquer, doing things separately when I have respite or when the kids have different days off school or time with their father? Putting everything through this filter means we only do the things we really want to do. There is no mindless joining in when so much effort must be made.

Families with a disabled family member are far more likely to experience financial difficulties, making days out, holidays and many activities not just physically challenging to arrange for but also extremely difficult to afford. We must all ask ourselves, is it worth it? And for many of the traditional and expensive activities, even if we know the person we are supporting would enjoy it, the answer may well often be no. This means we have to get creative about how we find joy and pleasure in our lives. This may require a lot more effort and quite a lot of letting go. But joy is available to us in so many surprising ways and sometimes a complete rethink about how we access it can allow us more than we imagined possible.

Small moments

Mary Susan McConnell (see Chapter 4, page 93) was reminded of this recently after her daughter had a severe seizure that had them in an ambulance for the first time in a long while. Leaving the house suddenly in the morning and not getting back till late that night, they arrived home in the dark. Although they were grateful to be home, they were shaken by the sudden change in Abiella's seizure activity after it had been stable for so long. As they opened the doors to the house, Mary Susan was greeted by lots of twinkling battery-powered candles. She remembered in that moment that she had put them on timers, to come on at dusk. It was such a cosy and joyful sight to come into on a winter's night, she said, after a long and trying day in the hospital. It reminded her that doing tiny things for ourselves can create so much joy on a tricky day. She went on to make a list of 75 small things that bring her joy, printed it out and stuck it on her fridge so that she remembered to do them regularly, whether she was feeling low and needed a pick-me-up, or just wanted a little more pleasure and fun in their lives. The list ranges from free sensory experiences like walking barefoot on grass, to wearing an item of clothing you usually save for 'best', to rearranging the furniture in a new and unexpected way. It was doing this one day that she discovered the immense joy of having a couch in the kitchen and they now eat together at a table in the dining room, leaving space in the kitchen for lounging around.

It might be easy to get caught up in the big things that we think will bring us joy, the big celebrations, holidays abroad, our kids reaching certain milestones. But for so many of us these big things might be impossible, unlikely or even bring huge amounts of distress. But what are these big things, if not many tiny moments put together? When we dissect what it is we are really searching for, then we are far more likely to find ways to access the pleasure and joy we are looking for. Small things such as listening to a favourite song, dancing in the kitchen, eating a delicious meal, enjoying a really good cup of coffee, allowing yourself the time to sit and read a book and wearing your favourite jumper, when woven throughout our day can bring immense joy with little effort. And life, after all, is made up of these days of tiny moments.

When you have limited time together

Amy Cooper and her family have found many ways over the years to find adventures, big and small. When Amy's daughter Rosa was 10 months old, she received a diagnosis that would change everything. Though they were aware she had developmental delays, a diagnosis of Canavan disease came with a life-limiting prognosis: the average life expectancy of a person with this rare genetic neurological condition is four to seven years old, though there are people around the world who have lived into early adulthood. With the knowledge that their time as a family was limited, Amy and her husband Gareth have put joy and fun at the centre of their lives. A few years ago they bought a camper van to create a safe and fun way to see more of the world. Along with Rosa and her little brother Ithan, they made trips to Italy, Scotland and France. Knowing that Rosa's medical needs would increase over time, they took advantage while they could. The van is familiar and comfortable for Rosa. In it they can stop as often as they need for her tube feeds, and if she needs to be changed. They can stay with friends or family or rent cottages when they arrive to create a comfortable base from which to explore.

Rosa is now 11 and has outlived her initial prognosis. Travelling has become a little more difficult; Amy was finding it was harder for her to recover from longer journeys, so they stick closer to home. From their home in Cornwall there are lots of wonderful destinations within a couple of hours that they are enjoying. She told me the decision to stick close to home has been quite liberating and no less fun. There can be a bit of pressure, she says, when there are a lot of choices. Rather than looking at everything they can't do, they have chosen to look at the things they can still do, and are making the most of it. Making the most of it certainly seems to be a quality the whole family are good at. Whether it's travelling or having cinema nights at home, or even the ceramics business that Amy built up at home so that she and Gareth can both be on hand with the kids, ready to drop everything if needed – everything they do as a family is designed to enjoy life with Rosa while they have the opportunity.

As the kids have grown, they have started to do more with Ithan on his own too. Amy and Gareth came to realise that Rosa didn't always want to do what her brother did, and vice versa. Gareth has started taking Ithan on surfing weekends and Amy is taking Rosa to a singing group that they both love. Last year they took their first trip to a festival without Rosa, while she spent a weekend in respite. Amy had been unsure how she would feel about it, but it turned out to be a wonderful and liberating weekend. Rosa had a great time where she was, and she and Gareth were able to give Ithan their full attention, with the freedom to roam about a festival for a whole weekend without any caring responsibilities. Though they want to do as much as possible together as a family, she said it was time to admit that that wasn't always what was best for the kids.

Travel

After a lifetime of travel, it has not been easy to adjust to the fact that this won't be a big part of my children's lives. My dad's work took us all over the world when I was a child, and that continued as I became an adult and lived and worked in a number of different countries. Although I was more than ready to slow down when I became pregnant with Arthur, I had never imagined I would be in a position where getting on a plane would be so distressing for him that it would be impossible for him to visit my family in Australia. It was one of the things that made me feel panicked in the middle of the night, far away from my family, thinking about how little my children would know of where I came from. A feeling of being trapped under an enormous weight that I couldn't throw off. But what exactly was it that I was worried about missing out on? Aside from seeing family and old friends back home, I decided it was necessary to figure out what it was that I imagined we would all gain from travel, and perhaps then find it in other ways. I thought back to what I got from my best travel experiences, and it always came back to a few things. Adventure, discovery, time with people I loved, and, paradoxically both a break from day-to-day routine and the creation of tradition and ritual. I became determined to figure out ways to bring this into our life as a family in creative and sometimes unusual ways.

For many reasons, going away from home can be extremely challenging for families with a disabled family member. The costs of finding somewhere suitably accessible – especially when you're already under financial strain from having to work reduced hours, or to give up work altogether – cannot be underestimated. Then if you rely on paid carers for support, going away can mean doing without them, making being away often more exhausting and stressful than being at home. Add to that the extra stresses of not having access to all your usual home comforts that make life for the person you're supporting easier, plus the planning for potential access problems and all the unknowns that a new environment can bring, and attempting trips becomes completely overwhelming and out of reach. But travel and holidays are a way to connect with each other and a chance to get away from school and therapy and work demands. A chance to experience new things. So how can we create a sense of adventure and connection without actually going away? With a little creativity, adventure is something we can find in our day-to-day lives.

A few years ago, between work, lack of support and lack of funds, it became clear we wouldn't be able to go away that summer. The seven weeks of summer holidays stretched ahead with nothing booked in. After feeling frustrated and despondent at first, I tried to think about what it was that I would want the three of us to be getting out of a trip away anyway. Adventure. We needed some sense of adventure, I thought, so I set about trying to create some.

Knowing how much Arthur had enjoyed the open fires of a trip to west Wales, I bought a metal fire pit for the garden. I called over the garden fence and invited the neighbours over to enjoy the fire with us. The kids cooked marshmallows on sticks and ran around our garden all evening, just as they would have done if we had been away from home. My Polish neighbour produced a cast-iron pot and, using a traditional recipe, created a camping dish she always had as a child, of bacon, potatoes and beetroot, cooked right on the fire. Arthur was mesmerised by the fire and smoke. When he needed to take breaks from everyone, he went into the house and back on his iPad for a time, before joining us again when he was ready. He was safe and comfortable in our house, so I could relax and enjoy the outdoors and the fire and friends without watching him like a hawk. As it got dark and the fire started to die down, I realised that it had been as much pleasure as the last time we had gone away, without any of the hard work. Friends, good food and drink, the outdoors, a fire. I knew then that although going away occasionally was still important, if we just got a bit creative, there was so much we could do right here at home.

That summer I also bought a hammock, which was one of the best decisions I have made. All of us could pile in it together, snuggling and laughing. Arthur could swing himself back and forth to self-regulate, Agnes and her friends piled on it to play games and I would sneak out there in the dying light after bedtime and watch the sun set, glass of wine in hand. The £100 it cost (including a stand) was much cheaper than a holiday and gave us endless pleasure that summer and beyond.

There are many ways to create a sense of adventure and a feeling of being on holiday without going away overnight. Amy Cooper's family hold cinema nights, where they set up a projector, make a huge comfy bed on the floor of the living room and all snuggle up together. If it's safe for everyone to do so, you could even camp there all night. Days out locally can be followed by picnics on the kitchen floor or in the back garden in the late evening sun, to draw out that feeling of being in holiday mode. Spend a little more than you usually would on buying some food and drink that make it extra special, or allow yourself to order some fancy takeaway that is usually out of budget (it's still a lot cheaper than going away!). For a huge treat you could book a house cleaner to come in and clean your home from top to bottom and change all the sheets and enjoy that room service feeling you get from being in a hotel, but without any of the hard work of going away. You could even pick or buy flowers to put in all the bedrooms.

Carving out the possibility to travel and go on holiday has still been important to me. It has taken some rethinking and adjusting of expectations. Adventures are possible, they may just look a lot different to what I initially expected. They tend to be short, only a few nights away at a time. That seems to be a good length of time for my son and means we can go away a few times a year because it isn't too expensive. The frequency is important. The years we have managed three separate short trips spaced out have really helped my son be open and excited about the idea of going away. So far, except for a trip when he was a baby, he hasn't been away from home for any more than three nights. Perhaps this will change in the future, as we experiment more and as his needs change.

I have some exciting ideas about the kind of travel my son might enjoy in the future. I wonder if, like me, he'll enjoy a sleeper train. A private cabin, a bunk bed and a picnic of food from home all make me think it's a possibility we could try. I think of all the beaches we could visit if this was possible. The warm seas of Europe and all the delicious gelato that we could eat, the water parks with slides he'd be desperate to go down. But for now we stick to British beaches and countryside rivers, cosy cabins, outdoor fires, camping with friends. Places he can be wild and free, get filthy, throw stones in rivers but also retreat to the iPad when it's all a bit much. Without having to worry about physical accessibility we have lots of options open to us of where we can stay. Our challenges have been around what will be safe and what will engage Arthur. So we stay away from cities and towns, which hold little interest for him, and focus on water and wild places. We holiday with friends so there are extra eyes on Arthur when I need to do anything that will take my eyes off him. At home he's relatively safe, but once out in unknown environments I must be extra vigilant to keep him safe. Another reason for the short trips; I can manage sustained vigilance for only so long before I long to get back to our known safe and relaxed environment.

Freedom

In her book *Joyful*, Ingrid Fetell Lee describes the different aspects of joy which reveal the connection between the feeling of joy and the world around us that creates that feeling. She calls our attraction to nature and wild spaces part of the aesthetic of freedom – that deep human desire for open spaces and the natural world which she believes has its roots in our desire to be free from constraints. 'Joy thrives on the alleviation of constraints,'[104] she writes. Arthur is certainly much more free when we are in wild spaces. At home, in the classroom and going about day-to-day life in a city, Arthur must conform to a certain degree. While at home he has as much freedom as I can manage, he would be pouring water down the walls and tipping flour down cracks in all the floorboards, given half the chance. There are constraints to being inside or even in a confined garden, where we have neighbours who, though they are extremely forgiving, don't love it when endless objects are hurled over the fence. But on wild, wide beaches, Arthur can watch sand fly from his outstretched hands, shout at the top of his lungs at the waves, twist and turn and spin, all without needing to be reined in or constrained in any way. Nature provides endless sensory stimulation that he seeks. Wind and waves, sand and stones, water that trickles and pours, sticks to poke mud with and trees that sway, mesmerising in the breeze. Liberation, found in nature.

In rustic cabins we can be free from worries about muddy feet and sticky fingers, too. Relaxed spaces that allow Arthur to enjoy the world just as he pleases. We can rent places in open fields, far from anyone else, not having to try to keep his noise down or worry about losing sight of him in crowds.

Though this wildness calls to me, we can get it in smaller ways close to home. In our corner of South London we are lucky to be surrounded by trees, overgrown Victorian cemeteries, parks and woods. Even our tiny and run-down garden, with the help of a hammock and fire pit, can give us the feeling of wildness. Our neighbour's large and overhanging apple tree and our small, young one provide a place to forage. A few old gutters, a cement tray and a hose make a water play corner, almost as satisfying to Arthur as a river. Access even to small amounts of green space can have an effect on our mental and emotional wellbeing. Studies show that those living in greener areas have less anxiety and depression and show more resilience in stressful life events than those who are in less green areas.[105] And a study of Alzheimer's patients has shown that access to garden spaces reduces the frequency of hostile outbursts which can be common as the diseases progresses.[106] This comes as no surprise to me. I can see the changes in Arthur as a natural space allows full expression of his movement and desire to interact with the world in ways that modern life does not allow him. As Ingrid Fetell Lee says: 'In nature, we find a temporary freedom from these constraints. In nature, anyone can have a full and free experience of the world.'

But joy is not just to be found in the natural world. In fact, it isn't just *found*. It can also be cultivated, created and savoured. And it is as much a part of the aesthetic world as it is in our relationships with one another. Reading Ingrid Fetell Lee's book was a reminder to me about how naturally in touch Arthur is with the sensory world and the joy that comes so easily to him from it. From floating objects like balloons and clouds, to rainbows on watery surfaces, brightly coloured walls, handfuls of tiny pompoms and repetitive harmonious patterns, Arthur shows me daily how easily accessible joy is, if only you are paying attention. Laura Godfrey, whose son Oscar has an undiagnosed genetic condition and who is also autistic (see Chapter 8, page 191), says that Oscar has made her look much more closely at the world around her. He is often transfixed and engrossed in the joys of the sensory world, making her stop and notice what she would have walked right past. I often wonder what the world looks like through my son's eyes. From the way he delicately sprinkles droplets of water down surfaces in utter delight, I can only imagine that he thinks the rest of us are mad for not paying proper attention to the world.

Looking back on videos of Arthur, it is clear that he has always paid more attention to the physical world than most. While he has struggled with shared attention, which is the focus of two people on an object or activity, he has never failed to make me question what *I* pay attention to. He may have mostly been dismissive of my attempts to get him to read a book or play with a toy, but if I paid enough attention I could see the things he finds more engaging in the world than conversation or a toy car.

Over the years his vocabulary has slowly grown but he still often struggles to give enough information to get across to me what it is he is referring to. One aspect of descriptive language that has become quite strong, though, is colour. Now whenever he is trying to tell me what he wants, he will refer to the colour of the object as the single most descriptive thing about it. A book about a dragon will be referred to as the 'yellow book', his iPad with its blue casing is always 'blue iPad' and his preferred ice cream is a Mr Whippy from a van which he calls 'white ice cream'. He separates smarties into coloured piles and enjoys pointing them all out before eating them in order. The sorting and the colours bring as much joy as the chocolate itself.

Celebrations

Like Mary Susan's list of things to bring peace and joy, I have my own growing mental list. That list has become important, because when the usual go-to things aren't accessible, then we must create our own. This has been important for travelling, as well as getting a sense of adventure while staying at home, but it has also been important when it comes to celebrations. Like many families with a disabled family member, we have to access celebrations in a slightly different way, so that they work for everyone. We have never spent a Christmas in Australia with my family and are unlikely to. That is something I have accepted. So instead of dwelling on what we can't do, I have had to work on the things we can do and create a joyful holiday celebration that embraces the fact we don't have family to spend it with. I decided instead to build a Christmas from scratch, all new traditions for our small family. We have a Christmas party every year at our house that we invite our local friends to. I can support Arthur much better in our house and he's happy having lots of people over, as long as he can stay close to me. The last couple of years I have invited other single mums to join us on Christmas day, so the kids get to enjoy some of the experience of having a busy family Christmas. If we can't always go out and about in the world to busy places that are too stressful for Arthur, or too stressful for me to keep him safe, then we create our own, right here at home. We can adapt everything to our needs here.

Having a real tree indoors is even more of a delight to Arthur than anyone else at Christmas. But it is prone to being pulled and tugged at and occasionally flung across the room with force. We pick the tree up about five times a day and redecorate each time. But with decorations made of felt and wood, nothing much is ever damaged, and it just gets a little messier as the days go by. As long as we are willing to embrace the mess of pine needles and wonky tree, Christmas is as much a delight in our house as any other. There is no letter to Santa, or anticipation of particular gifts. Sometimes I find just the right present that delights him so much he doesn't bother to open another gift till boxing day. Other times I miss the mark and everything but the chocolate coins and the bubbles in the stocking are completely ignored. It means that gifts are not the main aspect of Christmas for us. But the ritual and traditions of Christmas and other celebrations are important, even though we need to approach them a little differently. It punctuates the year and marks the passing of the seasons, anchoring us all as a family.

Large public firework celebrations are incredibly difficult for Arthur. Too crowded, too much waiting around for it to start. But the fireworks themselves he is utterly enthralled by. So we have our own firework display in the garden each year, Arthur with his ear defenders on, shouting 'rocket rocket rocket!' as they explode in starbursts of red and green and gold above our heads. As someone who grew up in a country where backyard fireworks are illegal, it never fails to delight me either. At Easter, he can take part in an egg hunt if his little sister helps him, showing him where she has found the brightly coloured mini eggs, hidden around the garden. Sometimes he doesn't want to do the searching and Agnes is very happy to collect them all and deposit them in his bucket. Birthdays aren't big parties but they have all the fun trappings that Arthur enjoys most. The cake and the candles that get blown out three times over, the balloons that get blown up and let go, flying around the room. A few gifts that may or may not hold much interest.

In her book, Ingrid Fetell Lee asks why the urge to celebrate is so strong in humans. When looked at in a purely rational way, it could be seen as a waste of energy and resources and hardly necessary to our survival. Certainly those of us who struggle to celebrate in the ways we were accustomed to, when the person we are supporting finds those celebrations too stressful or difficult to access, might be forgiven for giving up altogether. But celebration is an aspect of humanity that is universal across cultures and time. Whether it's the celebration of marriages, new life, harvests, the passing of another year or religious holidays, celebrations bring us together to create effervescent and collective joy. They don't need to be approached in the way everyone else does. And that can mean letting go of how we imagined things would be, which is not always easy. Whether it's accepting that a parent can no longer have a busy birthday celebration, and would be much happier with something quieter, or accepting that your child is going to be happier with a gift designed for a child many years younger than themselves, adjusting and adapting does not mean giving up. It means embracing all that is in front of you with full force and making the most of it.

Joyful aesthetics

With our minds filled with worries of access to health and social care and how we are going to pay our bills while supporting those who need a lot from us, it can be easy to ignore the small things designed to bring delight and unexpected joy. But tiny things add up to large amounts of positive emotions over time.

Ailbhe and Izzy Keane are sisters who are bringing some delight into an area that has largely been ignored. Izzy has spina bifida and has been a wheelchair user all her life. While Ailbhe was studying at design school, she had the idea to create a product that would improve the aesthetics of Izzy's wheelchair. Izzy has always seen her wheelchair as a source of freedom for her, and the fact they are so often dull-looking represented neither how it made her feel, nor her personality. Ailbhe created a brightly coloured wheel cover that reflected Izzy's outgoing nature. Izzy found that a decorated chair opened up positive conversations with others and gave her confidence while out and about. Seeing what a success they were, the sisters started collaborating with artists, designers and brands around the world, creating a large collection of designs as well as raising money for charity. Izzy Wheels has now won many national design awards in Ireland, and both sisters were named on the Forbes 30 Under 30 list in 2018.

Ailbhe says that the mission that drives Izzy Wheels is to challenge negative associations with wheelchairs and let users celebrate their individuality. They are joyful products, from bright geometric patterns, to botanical images and designs featuring people, whales, horses and donuts, with collaborations from artists such as Camille Walala, Mireia Ruiz, Bodil Jane and many more. They have even teamed up with Barbie to create an Izzy Wheels for the latest Barbie in a wheelchair. Wheelchairs are expensive and, for a relatively affordable price, the addition of an Izzy Wheels cover can completely transform the appearance.

Izzy says that Izzy Wheels is all about empowerment. To her, it takes the wheelchair beyond something functional and incorporates it into your sense of style. As a child, Izzy says that any time she saw wheelchairs on TV it was always accompanied by a sad story, and she didn't see anyone who had a positive relationship with their medical devices. She says: 'Something which always annoyed me was the message, "see the person, not the disability". You can see my wheelchair, there's nothing wrong with that and nothing wrong with you for seeing it.'[107] The strap line for the brand is: 'If you can't stand up, stand out.'

From beautiful mobility to aids, to brightly coloured clothing, to fresh cut flowers and homes bursting with natural light and cheerfully painted walls, it is easy to be dismissive of the power of joyful aesthetics to lift our mood. These small things added together can have a huge impact on how we experience the world. We don't always need to go out and spend money on these things. Sometimes it can be a matter of just noticing what is already around us and taking the time to savour it. Like Arthur showing me with delight the flock of birds that twist and swoop in patterns in the sky, or how droplets of water create magical patterns on glass. He is simply pointing out what is already there, waiting to be noticed.

Paying attention

As humans, something that has served us well on the evolutionary front is our strong negativity bias: that when of equal intensity, things of a more negative nature have a greater effect on our psychological state than neutral or positive things. But this same negativity bias that keeps us safe from harm by us easily being able to recall all the most difficult and worst things we encounter can mean that if we don't make an effort we can be fooled into think-ing the world is filled only with hardship, inequity and sorrow. If we pay attention we will realise how much joy is around us too. As we pay more attention to the things that delight us, we lay more pathways in our brain to notice and pay attention to those things in the future. With a little practice, we can all increase our joy spotting.

Savouring is something else we all know how to do; we just sometimes need to remind ourselves to do it. It can be an effort-less way to restore energy when we are feeling depleted and to remind ourselves of the good things that exist. That first cup of tea in the morning: instead of being hurriedly gulped, it can bring so much pleasure if we just take even a few extra seconds to savour the warmth, smell, taste and, quite frankly, that first hit of caffeine. We don't just have to savour food and drinks, though. When Suzy Reading (see Chapter 6, page 138) was supporting her father while also looking after her newborn, she would deliberately time a beach-side walk with her baby to coincide with a sunset, and savoured the view as long as she could. She describes savouring as a way to amplify and sustain enjoyment. It might be really enjoying a piece music or looking at a favourite flowering plant in the front garden every time you leave the house. You can also savour the past by recalling moments of deep enjoyment, and savour the future by anticipating and visualising an event you're looking forward to, like a holiday. It sounds small, but savouring can have a powerful effect on our mood.

Allowing yourself to experience joy

At 39 years old, Amy Cooper (see Chapter 10, page 229) had an opportunity to do something she'd been dreaming of since childhood. She started trapeze lessons. Although she no longer has the desire to run away with the circus, in the last few years she has begun performing with one. Circuses are places of delight. Sparkling costuming, daring aerial feats, music and spectacle, it is hard not to become child-like with wonder at them. Her children come and see her perform, and though Rosa doesn't vocalise often, Amy said that while she's on the trapeze she can hear noises of delight coming from her daughter. It's been a huge source of joy for Amy and something the whole family can enjoy too. Amy is certain that Rosa's prognosis is why they have been able to squeeze so much out of life. Though her condition puts limitations on them physically, it has opened up their world in other ways, making living in the moment and experiencing a deep sense of joy really accessible to them.

One thing that comes up again and again as I speak to families is that limitations, rather than reducing enjoyment and zest for life, can often do the opposite. Like Amy, Natalie Weaver's daughter Sophia (see Chapter 9, page 209) had a life-limiting diagnosis, and along with the discrimination they faced due to her facial differences, as well as her immune deficiency, there were many limitations on how they could experience the world together. But in the face of those limitations, Natalie chose to maximise all the joy she could. She made a promise to herself that Sophia's life, though it may be short and mostly spent at home, would be filled with love, fun and delight. She's proud of the fact she achieved this in Sophia's short ten-and-a-half years of life.

Though a life-limiting condition for the person we love and support may act as a sharp reminder to enjoy the life we have been given to the full, it is not the only way to access it. As Ingrid Fetell Lee reminds us in her book *Joy*, the drive we have towards joy is the drive towards life. Without joy, play, a sense of magic or celebration, we might be surviving but we aren't thriving. We must remember that joy is an essential part of life, and notice it, create it and savour it. Like Izzy's wheelchair, joy spills out towards others and starts conversations. It's infectious and spreads. In parks, small toddlers follow Arthur around while he plays, watching as he sprinkles sand down slides and flaps in delight at the patterns it creates, always curious about what kind of play excites him.

Joy, though, is often tinged with another emotion, especially when we know what we are experiencing is finite or someone is missing. On trips to museums and zoos alone with my daughter, though I delight in her company and the way she engages with the world, there is a sense in the background of someone missing. I know rationally Arthur is happier at his holiday club or with the babysitter than traipsing around a museum, but as a mother I can feel split in two, with that tinge of sadness colouring our activities. It was a similar feeling to when he started at his specialist school, in a different neighbourhood. An incredible school, with wonderful teachers, it is a place of great joy for both of us. But it came with letting go of being in a local school with his sister and being collected each day by me at the school gate. Years ago, this joy edged with sadness would frighten me, but I have learned that in order to embrace this life fully, I must meet and accept all the emotions that colour it. Amy doesn't know how long she will have Rosa, and though that affects every choice and decision they make, far from making her afraid to experience life, it has meant she has thrown herself into joy, knowing fully that what they have is finite.

Conclusion

'We think that the point is to pass the test or overcome the problem, but the truth is that things don't really get solved. They come together and they fall apart. Then they come together again and fall apart again. It's just like that. The healing comes from letting there be room for all of this to happen: room for grief, for relief, for misery, for joy.'[108]

Pema Chodron, author and Buddhist teacher

Over the course of writing this book, talking to other carers and reflecting on my own two different experiences, one thing has become clear to me. Though some people may wish the role of carer had never fallen on their shoulders, once you scratch beneath the surface it is clear that many do not feel this way at all. While there may be very difficult days for so many, the responsibility of supporting someone they love has given them a sense of purpose and pride, and a powerful realisation that they are capable and have the capacity for more than they ever knew.

That's not to say that most carers aren't desperate for more support; longing to feel less isolated; in dire need of more rest; and swallowed up by fears of a future when they may struggle to provide the same level of care. There is also the matter of the up to 700,000 young carers in the UK who do an estimated £12,000 worth of caring each year.[109] Caring which should be being provided by social services, not young children.

Many carers will be supporting their loved one right through until their death. Others, like myself and many of the parent carers I have spoken to, face a very different kind of fear. The knowledge that at some point in the distant future, we will die and someone else will have to take over the care of our child. It is a deep fear that when spoken of can make even the calmest parent panic – because there is no way to answer the question of who will care for a disabled child once their parents have died. Learning to live with that uncertainty is perhaps the best we can do. Taking life one step at a time, one milestone at a time. I don't dwell further into the future than the next few years. Just like I didn't know how I would manage to support a non-speaking ten-year-old when I had a newly diagnosed three-year-old, I know now that I have the capacity to learn, to find new solutions, to adapt to my son's changing needs. I have to believe that I will continue to adapt well into the future, whatever that might look like, and that solutions to the big questions will present themselves in time.

It is our collective responsibility as a society to care for the carers. It should not be up to each individual to move heaven and earth for their loved one, only to receive nothing themselves, and becoming depleted and feeling used up by a culture that would rather not see and hear the difficulties that caring can bring. As end-of-life doula Anna Lyons says, there needs to be a pyramid of care, with the cared for at the top, the carers underneath them, and a layer of support under the carers.

Illness, old age, disability and death are parts of life we have little control over. But in this age of advancing medicine we can be lulled into the idea that this isn't so. We pretend to ourselves that we can fix anything, that we can control what happens to us. Part of caring is about letting go of that control. Instead of asking ourselves, 'how do I fix this?' we can ask, 'how can I respond to this?' Can we also have the courage to ask ourselves, 'how do we make the best of this?'

We don't have to feel good about our role all the time in order to gain perspective from it, to have our hearts expanded by it and to even feel grateful for it. The act of supporting another person can reveal so many paradoxes. The depth of love alongside incredible loneliness. The heavy sense of duty mixed with a fulfilment that's greater than any we may have known before. Feelings of bitterness entangled with great tenderness. Heartache over losses and joy over seemingly tiny gains. These can all be true at once.

My daughter Agnes now walks a similar path to the one I walked as a teenager, that of the young carer. Though our situations are very different and she never has the sole care of responsibility for her brother, she has had to adapt and fit her life around Arthur's needs. Since she was tiny she has had to do more waiting, practise more patience and accept more compromise than most children her own age. She has eaten her dinner hidden under the table during violent meltdowns, abandoned playgrounds mid-adventure and learned to accept that her brother comes first at bedtime and other tricky transition times of the day. She has seen me cry in despair more times than I like to admit, and it is in those moments that I have worried about her. Not because having a disabled brother is so difficult but through having a mother who is too stretched, too tired and so close to the edge of what I can cope with.

But when I look back at my own experiences, though I desperately wish things had been different for my mum, I cannot say that I regret what I learned on the really difficult days. I would not have had the courage to live as I have or to be the parent my children have needed me to be without those experiences. I know that Agnes is already affected by her brother in the most positive ways. I can hear it in her voice as she explains autism to new friends in the park, in the way she talks openly about disability and her incredulity at any perceived infringements on her brother's rights of access. She does not passively accept she must come second, but understands in ways beyond her years that equal does not mean the same, rather equal means each getting what we need. And we are all equal in our house.

As carers we must remind ourselves that when we have a strong feeling of wanting to give up and run away, we need to rest. When we are afraid, we need to figure out exactly what it is we are afraid of. When we are angry, we need a space to share and express that feeling, free of judgment. Above all, we need to ask for the help we need. We need to remember that we must use those skills we have so finely tuned to advocate for ourselves too. We need a community around us, willing to provide this help for us. A community made up of family and friends, fellow carers and professionals. We also need the wider community to support us through making the world a more accepting and accessible place for all. Sharing our stories is one way we can create that community that is so needed. Stories that remind us that caring is as much a part of life as falling in love or having children or burying those we love. It is through our stories that we will remember that we are not alone.

Resources

Picture books which include disabilities

Just Because, Rebecca Elliott, Lion Hudson, 2018
Sometimes, Rebecca Elliott, Lion Hudson, 2011
Mama Zooms, Jane Cowen-Fletcher, Scholastic, 1993
It's Okay To Be Different, Todd Parr, Little, Brown and Company, 2001
I Love You Natty, Mia and Hayley Goleniowska, Downs Side Up, 2014
When Charley Met Emma, Amy Webb, Beaming Books, 2019
Hiya Moriah, Victoria Nelson, Koehler Kids, 2019
Eli, Included, Michelle Sullivan, 2019
Freddie and the Fairy, Julia Donaldson, Macmillan Children's Books, 2011
Dachy's Deaf, Jack Hughes, Wayland, 2013
What Happened to You?, James Catchpole, Faber, 2020
The Adventures of Kenzie-Moo, Tanya Savva, Little Wing Books, 2018

On childhood bereavement

The Magical Wood, Mark Lemon, Lemon Drop Books, 2018

For older kids

Department of Ability, comic book available at www.departmentof ability.com
Not So Different, Shane Burcaw, Roaring Brook Press, 2017

Books by disabled writers

The Reason I Jump, Naoki Higashida, Sceptre, 2014
Fall Down 7 Times, Get Up 8, Naoki Higashida, Sceptre, 2018
Loud Hands, Julia Bascom, Autistic Self Advocacy Network, 2012
If at Birth You Don't Succeed, Zach Anner, Macmillan USA, 2017
The Pretty One, Keah Brown, Atria Books, 2019
Say Hello, Carly Findlay, HarperCollins AU, 2019
Laughing at My Nightmare, Shane Burcaw, Square Fish, 2016
Strangers Assume My Girlfriend is My Nurse, Shane Burcaw, First
    Second, 2019
The World I Fell Out Of, Melanie Reid, Fourth Estate, 2019
Pride Against Prejudice, Jenny Morris, The Women's Press, 1991
I Might Be You, Barb Rentenbach and Lois Prislovsky, 2012
Neurodiversity, Barb Rentenbach and Lois Prislovsky, 2016
A Short History of Falling, Joe Hammond, Fourth Estate, 2019
Typed Words, Loud Voices, Amy Sequenzia, Autonomous Press,
    2015
Aspergirls, Rudy Simone, Jessica Kingsley Pub, 2010
Resistance and Hope, Alice Wong, Disability Visibility Project, 2018

Charities

There are many hundreds of charities that support people with specific disabilities and their carers. The following aim to support and represent *all* disabled people and unpaid carers.

UK

Carers UK: www.carersuk.org – help and advice for carers, campaigns
    and more
Carers Trust: www.carers.org – support and advice for carers
Scope (the Disability Equality Charity of England and Wales): www.
    scope.org.uk – practical information, support and campaigning for
    a fairer society
Contact a Family: www.contact.org.uk – for families with disabled children
Disability Rights UK: https://www.disabilityrightsuk.org/ – Disabled
    people leading for change, working for equal participation for all

Disability Information Scotland: http://www.disabilityscot.org.uk/ – Providing up to date information for disabled people in Scotland

Disability Action: https://www.disabilityaction.org/ – A Northern Ireland charity working for a more inclusive society

Disability Wales/Anabledd Cymru: http://www.disabilitywales.org/ – Striving for the equality and rights of all disabled people in Wales

Ireland

Family Carers Ireland: https://familycarers.ie/ – Support, advice and services for family carers

Disability Federation of Ireland: https://www.disability-federation.ie/ – Making Ireland fairer for people with disabilities

Australia

Children and Young People with Disabilities Australia: https://www.cyda.org.au/ – CYDA's purpose is to advocate systemically at the national level for the rights and interests of all children and young people with disability living in Australia as individuals, members of a family and their community.

People with Disability Australia (PWDA): https://pwd.org.au/ – a national disability rights advocacy and representative organisation that is made up of, led, and governed by people with disability.

Carers Australia: https://www.carersaustralia.com.au/ – working to improve the health, wellbeing, resilience and financial security of carers and to ensure that caring is a shared responsibility of family, community and government.

The Carers Foundation: https://www.thecarersfoundation.org/ – providing wellness programs for carers (including young carers) to help relieve stress and burnout.

New Zealand

Disabled Persons Assembly NZ: http://www.dpa.org.nz/ – DPA New Zealand is a Disabled Person's Organisation (DPO) that includes all disability groups. They work in collaboration with others to achieve inclusion for all New Zealanders.

Carers New Zealand: http://carers.net.nz/ – A national charity for family carers in New Zealand providing resources, information and support, as well as campaigning for carers rights

Self-Compassion

https://self-compassion.org/ – Dr Kristin Neff's website, which is full of resources for practicing self-compassion and central point to find a teacher where you live

https://chrisgermer.com/ – Chris Germer's website which has free resources such as guided meditations

Mindfulness Apps

Calm App: https://www.calm.com/ – Calm is one of my favourite mindfulness apps. It has meditations starting from just 3 minutes, including Loving Kindness, as well as body scans, less guided choices and beginner guides. It also has a whole host of options for helping with sleep and masterclasses on self-compassion and gratitude.

Headspace: https://www.headspace.com/ –Headspace is another leading mindfulness app that can teach you how to mediate, has lots of bite-sized mediations as well as articles and videos that teach various mindfulness techniques as well as plenty about improving sleep.

Insight timer: https://insighttimer.com/ – Insight Timer is a free app with thousands of meditations available from mindfulness teachers around the world. It's a less curated app but it is possible to save your favourites and it's completely free.

Other useful resources

www.self-compassion.org – Dr Kristin Neff's website which contains free resources for practising self-compassion

If you urgently need someone to listen or are in a crisis, helplines are
   listed below:

UK and Ireland
Samaritans – call 116 123 (available 24hrs a day)
samaritans.org

Australia
Lifeline – call 13 11 14 (available 24hrs a day)
lifeline.org.au

New Zealand
Lifeline – 0800 543 354 (available 24hrs a day)
lifeline.org.nz

Bibliography

Daring Greatly, Brené Brown, Penguin Life, 2015
The Gifts of Imperfection, Brené Brown, Hazelden Publishing, 2018
Grief Works, Julia Samuel, Penguin Life, 2018
Being Mortal, Atul Gawande, Profile Books, 2015
NeuroTribes, Steve Silberman, Allen & Unwin, 2015
The Conscious Caregiver, Linda Abbit, Adams Media, 2017
The Mindful Path to Self-Compassion, Christopher Germer, Guilford Press, 2009
The Mindful Self-Compassion Workbook, Kristin Neff, Christopher Germer, Guilford Press, 2018
Teaching the Mindful Self-Compassion Program, Kristin Neff, Christopher Germer, Guilford Press, 2019
Pride Against Prejudice, Jenny Morris, The Women's Press, 1991
Crippled, Frances Ryan, Verso Books, 2019
Laughing at My Nightmare, Shane Burcaw, Square Fish, 2016
Strangers Assume My Girlfriend is My Nurse, Shane Burcaw, First Second, 2019
The Self-Care Revolution, Suzy Reading, Aster, 2017
A Burst of Light and Other Essays, Audre Lorde, Dover Publications, 2017
The How of Happiness, Sonja Lyubomirsky, Piatkus, 2010
Stumbling on Happiness, Daniel Gilbert, Harper Perennial, 2007
Burnout, Emily Nagoski and Amelia Nagoski, Vermillion, 2019
The Power of Meaning, Emily Esfahani Smith, Rider, 2017
Resilient, Rick Hanson, Rider, 2018

Not What I Expected, Rita Eichenstein, Perigee Books, 2015

A Manual For Heartache, Cathy Rentzenbrink, Picador, 2017

The Pursuit of Happiness, Ruth Whippman, Windmill Books, 2016

Diversify, June Sarpong, HQ, 2019

How to Do Nothing, Jenny Odell, Melville House Publishing, 2019

Joyful, Ingrid Fetell Lee, Rider, 2018

Neurodiversity, Barb Rentenbach and Lois Prislovsky, 2016

The School of Life: An Emotional Education, Alain de Botton, Hamish Hamilton, 2019

Why We Sleep, Matthew Walker, Penguin, 2018

With the End in Mind, Kathryn Mannix, William Collins, 2019

Invisible Women, Caroline Criado Perez, Chatto & Windus, 2019

References

1 https://www.scope.org.uk/news-and-stories/coronavirus-bill/
2 Carers UK *State of Caring* report 2019, page 2
3 Papworth Trust, Disability Facts and Figures, 2018
4 https://www.carersuk.org/images/News__campaigns/The_world_Shrinks_Final.pdf
5 https://www.carersuk.org/news-and-campaigns/press-releases/facts-and-figures
6 Disability Rights, June 2013, Risk of major disability poverty rise, (Online), available at: https://www.disabilityrightsuk.org/news/2013/june/risk-major-disability-poverty-rise
7 Papworth Trust, Disability Fact and Figures, 2018
8 https://www.mckinsey.com/~/media/McKinsey/Featured%20Insights/Employment%20and%20Growth/How%20advancing%20womens%20equality%20can%20add%2012%20trillion%20to%20global%20growth/MGI%20Power%20of%20parity_Executive%20summary_September%202015.ashx
9 Carers UK, Facts About Carers, 2019
10 https://www.carersuk.org/images/Facts_about_Carers_2019.pdf
11 GP Patient Survey, 2018
12 Carers UK *State of Caring* report, 2019 , available at: http://www.carersuk.org /images / News__campaigns/CUK_State_of_Caring_2019_Report.pdf
13 *Ibid*
14 Carers UK *State of Caring Report*, 2019, available at: Dr Frances Ryan, *Crippled*, Verso Books, 2019

15 http://www.carersuk.org/images/News__campaigns/CUK_State_of_Caring_2019_Report.pdf

16 https://www.caregiver.org/caregiver-statistics-health-technology-and-caregiving-resources

17 Carers UK *State of Caring* report, 2019, available at: http://www.carersuk.org /images / News__campaigns/CUK_State_of_Caring_2019_Report.pdf

18 https://www.caregiver.org/caregiver-statistics-demographics

19 https://www.carersuk.org/news-and-campaigns/news/unpaid-carers-save-the-uk-132-billion-a-year-the-cost-of-a-second-nhs

20 https://catapult.co/stories/what-the-world-gets-wrong-about-my-quadriplegic-husband-and-me

21 Brené Brown, *Daring Greatly*, Penguin Life, 2015

22 Alain De Botton, *The School of Life: An Emotional Education*, Hamish Hamilton, 2019

23 Brené Brown, *The Gifts of Imperfection*, Hazelden Publishing, 2018

24 *Ibid*

25 https://www.theguardian.com/society/2019/jun/26/social-care-funding-crisis-putting-tens-of-thousands-at-risk

26 Brené Brown, *Daring Greatly*, Penguin Life, 2015

27 https://adiaryofamom.com/faqs/

28 Barb Rentenbach and Lois Prislovsky, *Neurodiversity*, 2016

29 https://www.gov.uk/definition-of-disability-under-equality-act-2010

30 https://catapult.co/stories/what-the-world-gets-wrong-about-my-quadriplegic-husband-and-me

31 Jenny Morris, *Pride Against Prejudice*, The Women's Press, 1991

32 http://suburbanautistics.blogspot.com/2017/10/grief-isnt-natural-its-product-of.html

33 Barb Rentenbach and Lois Prislovsky, *Neurodiversity*, 2016

34 Shane Burcaw, *Strangers Assume My Girlfriend is My Nurse*, First Second, 2019

35 Stella Young Ted Talk: https://www.youtube.com/watch?v=8K9Gg164Bsw

36 Papworth Trust, Disability Facts and Figures, 2018

37 *Ibid*

38 LeDeR Annual Report, 2018, available at: http://www.bristol.ac.uk/media-library/sites/sps/leder/LeDeR_Annual_Report_2018%20published%20May%202019.pdf

39 Shane Burcaw, *Strangers Assume My Girlfriend is My Nurse*, First Second, 2019

40 Cheryl Strayed, *Brave Enough*, Atlantic Books, 2015

41 Rita Eichenstein, *Not What I Expected*, Perigree Books, 2015

42 http://www.autreat.com/dont_mourn.html

43 https://www.merriam-webster.com/dictionary/grief

44 Rita Eichenstein, *Not What I Expected*, Perigree Books, 2015

45 Daniel Gilbert, *Stumbling on Happiness*, Harper Perennial, 2007

46 Sonja Lyubomirsky, *The How of Happiness*, Piatkus, 2010

47 Medvec V.H. et al (1995), 'When less is more: counterfactual thinking and satisfaction among Olympic medalists', *Journal of Personality and Social Psychology, 69 (4) 603–10 PMID*

48 Solnick, S.J., & Hemenway, D. (1998), 'Is more always better?: A survey on positional concerns', *Journal of Economic Behavior & Organization, 37(3), 373–383.*

49 Koo, M. Algoe, S.B., Wilson, T.D., Gilbert, D.T. (2008), 'It's a wonderful life: mentally subtracting positive events improves people's affective states, contrary to their affective forecasts', *Journal of Personality and Social Psychology, 95(5), 1217*

50 Rick Hanson, *Resilient*, Rider, 2018

51 Emmons, R.A. and McCullough, M.E. (2003), 'Counting blessings vs burdens: an experimental investigation of gratitude and subjective wellbeing in daily life', *Journal of Personality and Social Psychology, 84, 365–376*

52 Emily and Amelia Nogoski, *Burnout*, Vermilion, 2019

53 Sonja Lyubomirsky, *The How of Happiness*, Piatkus, 2010

54 Tedeschi, R.G., Park, C.L. and Calhoun, L.G. (Eds). 'Post traumatic growth: Positive changes in the aftermath of crisis', Lawrence Erlbaum Associates Publishers, 1998

55 Sonja Lyubomirsky, *The How of Happiness*, Piatkus, 2010

56 Julia Samuel, *Grief Works*, Penguin Life, 2018

57 L.R. Knost

58 https://thebaffler.com/latest/laurie-penny-self-care

59 Audre Lorde, *A Burst of Light*, Dover Publications, 2017

60 Carers UK State of Caring Report, 2019, availble at: http://www.carersuk.org/images/News__campaigns/CUK_State_of_Caring_2019_Report.pdf

61 Papworth Trust, Disability Facts and Figures, 2018

62 https://www.ons.gov.uk/employmentandlabourmarket/

peopleinwork/earningsandworkinghours/articles/womenshoul-dertheresponsibilityofunpaidwork/2016-11-10

63 Emily and Amelia Nogoski, *Burnout*, Vermilion, 2019

64 Matthew Walker, *Why We Sleep*, Penguin, 2018

65 Emily and Amelia Nogoski, *Burnout*, Vermilion, 2019

66 Green, K.M., B.J. Anderson et al. (2003), 'Warm Partner Contact Is Related to Lower Cardiovascular Reactivity,' *Behavioural Medicine 29 123–130*

67 https://www.helpguide.org/articles/mental-health/laughter-is-the-best-medicine.htm

68 https://www.ncbi.nlm.nih.gov/pmc/articles/PMC4035568/

69 Suzy Reading, *The Self-Care Revolution*, Aster, 2017

70 https://www.health.harvard.edu/healthbeat/writing-about-emotions-may-ease-stress-and-trauma

71 Neff, K. D. (2003). Self-compassion: An Alternative conceptualisa-tion of a healthy attitude toward oneself. *Self and Identity, 2*, 85–102

72 Neff, K. (2003), 'Development and Validation of a Scale to Measure Self-Compassion,' *Self and Identity, 2; 223-250*

73 Fresnics, A. and Borders, A. (2016), 'Angry Rumination Mediates the Unique Associations Between Self-Compassion and Anger and Aggression', *Mindfulness 8(3), 554–564*

74 Diedrich, A., Burger, J., Kirchner, M., Berking, M. (2016), 'Adaptive emotion regulation mediates the relationship between self-compassion and depression in individuals with unipolar depression', *Psychology and Psychotherapy; Theory, Research and Practice, 90(3) 247–263*

75 Hollis-Walker & Colosimo (K. (2011). Mindfulness, Self compas-sion and happiness in non-meditators: A theoretical and empirical examination. *Personality and Individual Differences, 50*, 222–227

76 Dr K Neff and Dr C Germer, *The Mindful Self-Compassion Workbook*, Guilford Press, 2018

77 Sirois, F.M (2014). 'Procrastination and Stress: Exploring the role of self-compassion,' *Self and Identity*, 13(2), 128-145

78 Patzak, A., Kollmayer, M. & Schober, B. (2017) 'Buffering imposter feelings with kindness; The mediating role of self-compassion between gender-role orientation and the imposter phenomenon,' *Frontiers in Psychology*, 8, 1289

79 Neff, K. D., Hsieh, Y. & Dejitterat, K. (2005). 'Self-compassion, achievement goals and coping with academic failure,' *Self and Identity*, 4, 263-287

80 Neely, M. E., Schallert, D. L., Mohammad, S. S., Roberts, R. M., & Chen, Y. (2009). 'Self-Kindness when facing stress: The role of self-compassion, goal regulation, and support in college students' wellbeing,' *Motivation and Emotion*, 33, 88-97

81 Breines, J. G., & Chen, S. (2012). 'Self-compassion increases self-improvement motivation,' *Personality and Social Psychology Bulletin*, 38(9), 1133-1143

82 Duckworth, A. (2016) *Grit: The power of passion and perseverance*. Simon & Schuster

83 Neff, K. D. & Beretvas, S. N. (2013), 'The role of self-compassion in romantic relationships,' *Self and Identity*, 12(1), 78-98

84 Lloyd, J., Meurs, J., Patterson, T. G., & Marczak, M. (2018). 'Self-compassion, coping strategies, and caregiver burden in caregivers of people with dementia,' *Clinical Gerontologist*, 42(1), 47-59.

85 Neff, K. D., & Faso D. J. (2014). 'Self-compassion and wellbeing in parents of children with autism,' *Mindfulness*, 6(4), 938-947

86 Dr K Neff and Dr C Germer, *The Mindful Self-Compassion Workbook*, Guilford Press, 2018

87 Wagner, D. Schneider, D. J. Carter, S.R. & White T. L. (1987), 'Paradoxical effects of thought suppression', *Journal of Personality and Social Psychology 53(1),* 5-13

88 Dr K Neff and Dr C Germer, *The Mindful Self-Compassion Workbook*, Guilford Press, 2018

89 www.self-compassion.org

90 Sylvia Plath, *The Bell Jar*, Faber & Faber, 2005

91 https://www.carersuk.org/images/News__campaigns/The_world_Shrinks_Final.pdf

92 *ibid.*

93 https://www.leonardcheshire.org/about-us/press-and-media/press-releases/online-disability-hate-crimes-soar-33

94 https://publications.parliament.uk/pa/cm201719/cmselect/cmpetitions/759/75905.htm#_idTextAnchor015

95 Jaron Lanier, *Ten Arguments For Deleting Your Social Media Account Right Now*, Bodley Head, 2018

96 Dr Frances Ryan, *Crippled*, Verso Books, 2019

97 Cathy Rentzenbrink, *A Manual for Heartache*, Picador, 2017

98 Rick Hanson, *Resilient*, Rider, 2018

99 Emily Esfahani Smith, *The Power of Meaning*, Rider, 2017

100 Ruth Whippman, *The Pursuit of Happiness*, Windmill Books, 2016

101 Baumeister, R.F., Vohs, K.D., Aaker, J.L., Garbinksy, E.N. (2013), 'Some key differences between a happy life and a meaningful life', *The Journal of Positive Psychology 8, no. 6; 505–16*

102 Huta, V., Ryan, R.M. (2010), 'Pursuing pleasure or virtue; the differential and overlapping well-being benefits of hedonic and eudaimonic motives', *The Journal of Happiness Studies 11, no. 6*

103 Ingrid Fetell Lee, *Joyful*, Rider, 2018

104 Van den Berg A.E. et al (2010), 'Green Space as a buffer between stressful life events and health', *Social Science and Medicine 70(8); 1203–210*

105 Kuo F.E., Sullivan W.C. (2001), 'Aggression and violence in the inner city: Effects of Environment via Mental Fatigue', *Environment and Behaviour 33(4): 543–71*

106 https://www.thesun.ie/fabulous/4192438/irish-woman-changing-perceptions-disabilities/

107 Pema Chodon, *When Things Fall Apart*, Element Books, 2007

108 www.theguardian.com/commentisfree/2020/feb/27/child-labour-boris-johnson-migration-policies

Acknowledgements

Firstly, and most importantly, I'd like to thank every one of the interviewees who agreed to speak to me about their experiences. Most of them responded to an email without knowing anything about me and I will be forever grateful that they decided I could be trusted with their story. For each story mentioned in this book, there is a far larger story, so large and full in fact, that entire books could be written about each person. What has been included here is only a tiny portion of their rich and varied lives. Though in some cases I have made only passing reference to people, each conversation I had, had a huge impact on me personally and what I chose to focus on in this book. Each conversation opened up a world and a perspective that I will always treasure. Every one of you made this book an absolute pleasure to write. Special thanks to my dear friend Lucy Rogers, whose conversation over a glass of wine about difficult things really sparked the whole project off.

As this book began its life, I had a huge amount of support from a number of women I admire greatly. Thanks so much to Annie Ridout, Jen Carrington, Doreen Walton, Anna Whitehouse, Michelle Kane, Natasha Lunn, who each in their own way, whether through cheerleading, early reading, or encouraging my writing, helped see this book come to life.

Enormous thanks to my agent Abigail Bergstrom, who from the moment we sat down to discuss the topic of caring, entirely understood both its enormous importance as well as the difficulties for me around writing about disability as a non-disabled person. Abigail has that wonderful combination of being fully focused on engaging stories as well as a desire to see the publishing world filled with rich diverse voices. She has been a guiding light and a great companion on this journey. So too has Megan Staunton, who is always quick to reply, quick to smile and always has the answers when I have needed them. They have both been an incredible sounding board and each offered their own unique and very much valued opinions to the book.

Huge thanks to my editor Hannah Black for allowing me enormous freedom to write the book exactly as I felt it needed to be written. Always there when I had a question, but giving me space to get on with it, however I felt was best. It gave me the confidence I needed to get my head down and get the work done. It was a pleasure from start to finish.

Thanks also to the rest of the team at Coronet. To Sally Somers, for her excellent copy editing. Your perspective and expertise were most welcome. To Erika Koljonen, Jenny Platt and Helen Flood, all of whom have been carrying on heroically through changes never before seen as our society shuts down and the way in which we produce, promote and sell books has been completely turned on its head. Your hard work is so appreciated, as well as your vision for the book and those it will help.

Although you can see within the resources, the books by disabled authors that I recommend, I would also like to thank some specific writers, speakers and activists that have been absolutely vital to my education on disability and whose knowledge has made me a better feminist, mother and human. Whether it is on Twitter, podcasts, in books, on Instagram, Ted Talks, journalism or anywhere else, the following people have added a crucial perspective to my understanding of disability. Where possible, please buy their books, listen to their podcasts, hire them as writers and pay for them to speak at your events. Carly Findlay, Naoki Higashida, Keah Brown, Emily Ladau, Barb Rentenbach, Jenny Morris, Eliza Hull, Alice Wong, Shane Burcaw, Dan White, Christa Holmans, Mik Scarlet, Samantha Renke, Sara Gibbs, Sally Darby, Frances Ryan, Amit Patel, Amy Kavanagh, Sinead Burke, Nina Tame and the much missed Stella Young. Special thanks to Emma Fowler, whose Instagram chats have always been both a pleasure and life enhancing. And to Kieran Rose, whose unique perspectives encapsulated so many of the ideas I wanted to explore and whose help on this project I will always be grateful for. Thank you for trusting me and helping me share these ideas with the world.

To Hat Margolies for her patience and understanding as I took a massive step back from shooting to meet my writing deadlines. To Ruth and Andrew for endless cups of tea and cheery company. Thank you to all my local friends, who have always picked me up and supported me when I have no family to turn to. To Nico, Clare, Monica, Alex, Tracy, Sandra, Harriet, Fiona, Helen, Nena, Velia, Gill and Asia who have all rescued me at one time or another. Thanks also to Haresh Patel for all his support with the kids.

To my dad Simon and my brothers Ash and Pip, for supporting my decision to write about Mum and giving me free reign to do it however I pleased. This is your story too and I know we each had different experiences. I love you all so much. I wish I wasn't so far away.

Marisa, my best friend and the love of my life. Where would I be without you? I will forever be grateful we found each other at uni all those years ago. Thank you for allowing me to share a tiny bit of our friendship with the world.

There is one person for whom this book could actually not have been written without. Thank you to our wonderful nanny Julie for being there for my children, for everything you contribute to our home and for the love you bring to work with you. You have rescued me from the brink so many times and I couldn't be the mother I am without you.

And to Ruairi, who has shown me that there are people in the world who are not afraid to choose a more difficult path, who choose love, rather than ease. The moments we get alone together are so precious and few and as I ploughed most of that time into working on this book, you showed me nothing but encouragement and support. I love you so much.